Nature

as Teacher

and Healer

NATURE
AS TEACHER
AND HEALER

*How to Reawaken
Your Connection with
Nature*

JAMES A. SWAN, PH.D.

Villard Books
New York
1992

All rights reserved under International and Pan-American
Copyright Conventions. Published in the United States by
Villard Books, a division of Random House, Inc.,
New York, and simultaneously in Canada by
Random House of Canada Limited,
Toronto.

Villard Books is a registered trademark of Random House, Inc.

Grateful acknowledgment is made to the following
for permission to reprint previously published
material:

NORTH POINT PRESS: Excerpt from "The Gifts" by Richard K.
Nelson, from *On Nature*, edited by Daniel Halpern. Copyright
© 1986 by Antaeus, New York, N.Y. Published by North
Point Press and reprinted by permission.

OHIO UNIVERSITY PRESS/SWALLOW PRESS: Excerpt from the
foreword by Lama Angarika Govinda in *Cuchama and
Sacred Mountains* by W. Y. Evanz-Wentz. Copyright
© 1981 by Ohio University Press/Swallow Press, Athens.

PAT LITTLE DOG: Excerpts from *The God Chaser* by
Pat Ellis Taylor. © Pat Ellis Taylor.

SHAMBHALA PUBLICATIONS, INC.: Excerpt from *Shadow and
Evil in Fairy Tales* by Marie-Louise von Franz, © 1974.
Reprinted by arrangement with Shambhala Publications,
Inc., P.O. Box 308, Boston, Mass. 02117.

Library of Congress Cataloging-in-Publication Data

Swan, James A.
Nature as teacher and healer / p. cm.
Includes bibliographical references and index.
ISBN 679-73879-7
1. Nature—Psychological aspects. I. Title.
BF353.5.N37S83 1992
155.9'1—dc20   91-21260

Manufactured in the United States of America
9 8 7 6 5 4 3 2
First edition

For Roberta and Andrew,
whose patience and support
have been invaluable.

NOTE: A percentage of the author's profits from the sale of this book goes to support work preserving the priceless heritage of traditional cultures and the ecosystems that support them.

NOTE: The self-help suggestions and techniques described in this book are in no way meant to replace professional medical assistance.

ACKNOWLEDGMENTS

The ideas presented in this book have been influenced by many people. My father, Donald Swan, was my first nature teacher. His initial guidance established a root that enabled me to realize how nature can be a source of knowledge and health. Bill Stapp has also had a great influence on my appreciation for nature and has given me many opportunities to grow, for which I'm extremely thankful.

I'm especially grateful to Rolling Thunder, Bill Fields, and Vine Deloria, Jr., for their guidance about Native American psychology and spiritual practices; to Stanley Krippner for helping me gain important insights into shamanism and parapsychology; and to Donald Michael for his insights into the psychology of social transformation. Several dinner conversations with Joseph Campbell helped bring things into perspective in a fashion that only Joe could do—may his spirit never die. Thanks also go to Mark Satin at *New Options* newsletter, Pat Ellis Taylor, Master Thomas Yun Lin, and Marie-Louise von Franz, for allowing me to reprint their work.

Support for projects reported in this book that have enabled my synthesis of this material has come from many sources including: the National Audubon Society Expedition Institute, the Institute for the Human Environment, the Government of American Samoa, the California Institute of Integral Studies, *Shaman's Drum* magazine, Joshua Mailman, the Beldon Fund, Laurance Rockefeller, the L. G. and Mary C. Skaggs Foundation, and the National Endowment for the Humanities.

Special thanks also go to Diane Reverand and Tom Fiffer at Villard Books and to my agent, Linda Allen, a gifted guide for writers through the wilderness of the literary world.

Throughout the process of living and writing this book, my wife, Roberta, and my son, Andrew, deserve far more credit than can be expressed in words for their patience, support, and love.

Finally I must pay my respects to the creatures of all the families of the nature kingdom for sharing their wisdom with me. When these pages reveal magic, it is theirs more than my own.

CONTENTS

INSIDE-OUT
ECOLOGY

*Nature is prime: it is there at birth;
society is next: it is only a shaper
of Nature, and a function moreover,
of what it shapes; whereas Nature is as
deep and, finally, inscrutable
as being itself.*

—JOSEPH CAMPBELL
The Flight of the Wild Gander

A cold drizzle was falling on the morning of September 20, 1990, as one hundred or so people assembled at the Chapin Mesa amphitheater in Mesa Verde National Park. They had come to this half-circle of stone seats carved into the lip of a quarter-mile-deep sandstone canyon to hear three speakers talk about Native American sacred places and the law. I had organized this third annual "Spirit of Place" symposium, so everyone looked at me to see if the session would be canceled.

I was about to say, "Maybe we should call it off," when Bill Tallbull, a barrel-chested Northern Cheyenne spiritual leader who was scheduled to be the second speaker, spoke up.

"Anyone got a cigarette?" Bill asked. We thought he wanted a smoke, and someone produced one. But instead of lighting up, Bill took the cigarette and walked off into the bushes, pulling the paper off. A few seconds later we heard a melodic chant and saw Bill's hand raised up above the bushes, tossing the tobacco to the four directions, the world below, the world above, and the center. A subtle sense of the extraordinary seemed to well up in all of us, creating a feeling of excitement, and people's spirits began to rise.

Two minutes later Bill emerged with a twinkle in his eye and said, "Let's wait a few minutes to see if there's any change. It's a long way to come from the Bighorn Medicine Wheel in Wyoming to Mesa Verde to be rained out."

Suddenly a giant form appeared over the amphitheater, a turkey vulture flying no more than fifty feet from the ground. Then another and another. In less than three minutes twenty-two of these cousins of the condor soared over us—in a perfect line. As the last vulture vanished from sight, with a rush of wings a flock of at least one hundred tiny golden-crowned and red-crowned kinglets landed in the pinyon pines around the amphitheater, singing excitedly. Something special was definitely in the air.

As if on cue, the dark rain cloud that had been looming stopped in its tracks and started to slide to the opposite side of the canyon. The rain stopped. I looked at my watch. It was 10:00 A.M., time for the program to begin. I walked onto the stage and introduced the first speaker, Evelyn Martin from the American Planning Association. As she began reading her paper, the sun came out, but only in the immediate vicinity of the amphitheater. As Evelyn talked, I noticed Bill Tallbull's lips moving slowly and silently. The dark cloud, now on the far side of the canyon, seemed stationary, and the wind had stopped blowing.

Half an hour later Evelyn finished, and now it was Bill's turn. His talk was about the work of the Medicine Wheel Alliance to save the Bighorn Medicine Wheel, an ancient circle of wise stones perched at 9,640 feet on the shoulder of Medicine Mountain not far from Sheridan, Wyoming. The stones are oriented to the sun and to the stars Aldebaran, Sirius, and Rigel—an American equivalent of Stonehenge. As Bill focused on his talk, I noticed the rain cloud across the canyon slowly inching toward us. Half an hour later the cloud was nearly overhead. Just as Bill said, "Thank you very much," a gust of wind swept through the amphitheater, dropping a sheet of rain. Spontaneously the entire crowd went "Ooo," as it became apparent that Bill's prayers had been holding the rain off. Soon everyone was running for cover, and the shower washed out the rest of the morning's speakers.

Our Current Predicament

The United States Environmental Protection Agency (EPA) reports that in 1989 U.S. industries poured 4.57 billion pounds of chemicals into the nation's air, water, and soil. More than eight hundred contaminants have been found in Great Lakes water, and the groundwater in at least thirty-eight states is tainted by pesticides.

Worldwide the consequences of environmentally damaging human activity on Mother Earth include global warming, acid rain, deforestation, the extinction of species at an unprecedented rate, famines, contamination of the entire biosphere, overpopulation, toxic buildups throughout the food chain, mountains of garbage, and decreasing supplies of mineral and energy resources. Thanks to the media and the collective efforts of Earth Day 1990, people today are more aware than ever before of the problems of the environment. There are success stories. Recycling has taken root across the country; once-careless companies are now trying to reduce environmental pollution; kids are planting trees and picking up litter. Yet, overall we seem to be losing ground rapidly.

To understand fully the ecological crisis, we must do more than treat its symptoms. We must acknowledge that all environmental problems originate in the human mind and manifest themselves as a result of human perceptions, attitudes, and decisions.

My professional discipline is environmental psychology—the study of the interaction between people and the world around them. Now that ecological concerns are finally being taken seriously, it sounds like an appropriate research area, but environmental psychology didn't even exist until the early 1970s. Prior to that time behavioral scientists had little to say about the influence of the physical environment on people's lives, unless it had to do with rats running through a laboratory maze or the conditions in a child's home. Even today there are only a few environmental psychologists, an indication of a great gaping hole in our understanding of human behavior. In contrast, traditional societies consider the link between people and nature as the primary force in shaping people's health and happiness. The bush psychology of shamans, wizards, witches, and witch doctors is largely concerned with how to strengthen the link between people and nature, and they have more success than we do at creating sustainable cultures. Perhaps the alchemical mind of a wizard is the ultimate key to helping us find answers to the ecological problems modern scientists can't seem to solve. What happened at Mesa Verde with Bill Tallbull and the rain cloud, I believe, was not a coincidence.

For the last twenty years I've been trying to understand how people in modern and ancient cultures relate to the environment. This quest has taken me from the broken-down inner city of Detroit, Michigan, to the sensuous golden-sand beaches—dotted with jet-black volcanic rocks—on the Manua Islands of American Samoa, from the corporate board rooms of major U.S. industries to the billiard-table-flat Arctic tundra on the Bering Sea, from the bowling-lane-like halls of the U.S. Department of Interior's headquarters in Washington, D.C., to the underground earthen ceremonial kivas of the Southwest Pueblo tribes, from psychiatric offices to shamanic rituals, and a lot of meetings with groups of mainstream Americans of many persuasions in between.

One thing I learned from these excursions is that one person's ecological nightmare may not present the slightest concern to another. In the late 1960s a paper plant along the Huron River in Ypsilanti, Michigan, made brightly colored papers from supposedly nontoxic dyes, which were subsequently dumped into the river after being used for each batch of paper. On various days the Huron River might be white, dark purple, blue, red, or yellow depending on the dyes used, and some people were up in arms about the situation, claiming the plant was polluting the water. Because the dyes weren't highly toxic, it was difficult to prove pollution was taking place, and in the midst of the debate, one woman wrote a letter to the Ypsilanti paper, thanking the company for their work. She said that she lived along the banks of the river and every morning she would go to the window first thing to see what beautiful color the river was that day!

BECOMING AN ENVIRONMENTALIST

Beauty may be in the eye of the beholder, but pollution damage increasingly can be documented with sophisticated scientific devices, as well as sensitivity to nature's moods, voices, and patterns. Regardless of how we conclude that something is wrong, all too often we wait until disaster strikes to show our ecological values, a dangerous game in a world where technology enables our actions to have such powerful consequences as Chernobyl, the Alaskan oil spill, or the eating away of the earth's protective ozone layer. We need to understand how to think ecologically and to act with as much passion to prevent eco-disasters as we use to rise to fight crises or show up for Earth Day rallies and concerts.

In the field of psychology Abraham Maslow revolutionized our understanding of human behavior when he realized that most of our theories of human behavior were based on studies of rats, chimpanzees, or mentally disturbed people rather than psychologically healthy people. To remedy this bias, Maslow studied people who were seemingly performing at levels of healthiness far exceeding norms, whom he called self-actualizing people.[1] Inspired by Maslow's work, I've been studying people who are dedicated ecologists, both famous and unknown, living and dead, in hopes of better understanding how to heal our split from harmony with nature and get us moving toward right eco-action. What emerges from this work are five general paths that lead up the mountain to becoming a committed supporter of nature.

One path to developing an ecological conscience is by absorbing and gathering information: reading, listening to radio shows and lectures, watching television, and relying primarily on secondhand reports from "expert" sources. As more and more people become aware in this way that we have an ecological crisis on our hands, their support for the environment swells, but it usually doesn't last. As Earth Day approached, ecology became the latest fad, but soon afterward interest in the environment as a national priority quickly dropped as more immediate issues like the war in the Persian Gulf and the economy took center stage.

I know only one leader in the environmental movement who feels he became deeply committed to mainstream environmental action through information exposure: Dr. Albert Baez, former director of education for the International Union for the Conservation of Nature and Natural Resources. A physicist and science educator, Al admits that his interest in conservation began with several friends—who were ardent conservationists for other reasons—urging him to start reading about ecology issues. The more he read, the more he became concerned, and eventually he switched his life's work from science education to conservation action.

A second path to becoming an environmentalist comes from having strong convictions about social justice. Many people who are moved by the spirit of Saint Augustine see environmental problems as just one more example of injustice resulting from the existing political and economic system. Often they are not ardent naturalists, and they may spend little time in natural areas. Nonetheless they are ready to throw themselves into ecological battles because they feel it's the right thing to do. Ralph Nader is a good example of someone becoming ecologically concerned because of a strong social conscience. So was the master organizer of social protest, Saul Alinsky. Some of the modern entertainers who have joined the ecology movement, such as Sting, Madonna, Jackson Browne, Martin Sheen, Jane Fonda, and Bob Geldof, also seem to see environmental activism as an extension of their concern for social justice.

The third path to developing deep ecological convictions involves personal confrontations with ecological problems that threaten personal health, property, or other species. Debra Dadd, who has become a world-recognized authority on toxic-free living, was forced to give up her career as a professional musician because she was chemically sensitive. Realizing that she would either have to figure out a way to live a chemically free life or die, she became an expert on living ecologically and found that she flourished in natural places, which kindled in her a new love for nature. Another is Fred Soyka, whose writing has done a great deal to inform the public of the health values of positive and negative air ions. Soyka's interest in air chemistry was triggered by his discovery that his long bout with a strange chronic physical and emotional sickness was due to his sensitivity to "something electrical about the air." Barry Commoner also seems to fall into this category; his initial interest in ecological issues was linked to fears about health effects of the fallout from atmospheric testing of nuclear devices. Farmworker union organizer Cesar Chavez's concern for pesticides also seems to fall within this motivational pathway to eco-activism.

The fourth path to ecological advocacy comes from an awareness of how health and fitness are linked to ecological quality. People on this path, such as organic-living champions John Robbins and the late Robert Rodale, feel strongly about the need to buy and eat organic foods, get more exercise, meditate or do yoga, and live and work in clean and safe environments. A visceral concern for ecological quality is much stronger and longer lasting than a purely cerebral one. Eating your way to ecological awareness may be a more effective way to establish an ecological conscience than being exposed to a media blitz, because you can feel the rightness of it in your body as well as knowing it in your head.

The fifth path is one that modern psychology has almost totally ignored, yet it is the most common and potent among all committed leaders of the ecological movement. Almost all the most dedicated ecologists can ultimately trace their passion to an almost mystical love for nature that arises from one or both of the following experiences: early positive encounters with nature, usually in the presence of loved adults, and later transcendental moments in natural places that may have had healing value. John Muir spent most of his boyhood in Scotland, then later in the woods of the Midwest escaping a tyrannical father. Ralph Waldo Emerson, Henry David Thoreau, and John Burroughs all felt that being alone in nature provided deep spiritual inspiration, like the Desert Fathers of the Christian tradition and the many Indian peoples seeking guidance on vision quests in solitude at sacred places. In his youth, folksinger Pete Seeger slipped into the woods alone and imagined himself as an Indian in perfect harmony with the animals and trees, laying the groundwork for a lifelong commitment to ecological action. Jacques Cousteau speaks with deep reverence of that transformational moment in his life when he made the first underwater descent with his invention, the aqualung. Rachel Carson's mother taught her biology out of doors, and later Carson found that retreating to remote ocean beaches renewed her, resulting in her beautiful book *The Sea Around Us.* The late Supreme Court Justice William O. Douglas was an ardent wilderness fighter, who linked his love for nature to a moment in his youth when his father died very unexpectedly. Standing beside the fresh grave in the prairie of eastern Washington State, Douglas felt a deep emptiness. He looked up at snowcapped Mount Adams and suddenly realized that his second father would be the mountain. Both David Brower and Loren Eiseley trace the origins of their fondness for nature to helping their ailing parents stay in touch with the world: Brower's mother went blind, and he had to become her "eyes"; Eiseley's mother was deaf, and as a result he developed a kind of sensory communication with her "which might have been conducted by the man-apes of the early ice age."

The common thread that unites all these people on this path is primal experiences with nature that result in feelings often verging on mystical rapture and awe. The major difference between people from traditional societies and members of modern society on this path is that older cultures plan for these alchemical experiences to occur in most or all members of the culture, while in the modern world they tend to happen rarely and almost always by accident. Further, once kinship bonding with nature has been established, traditional peoples have road maps and techniques for developing their roots in nature into health and personal power, whereas modern psychology questions the sanity of those who dare to voice their transcendent moments of nature kinship.

BONDING WITH NATURE

In science the term *concurrent validity* refers to a situation where two or more people using different research approaches arrive at the same conclusion, and it is considered an especially strong indication of a conclusion's truthfulness. Studying members of citizen environmental groups, professors Thomas Tanner and Harold Hungerford and their colleagues have concurrently concluded that the most committed environmental attitudes seem to arise from deep psychoemotional bonding experiences with nature. Many more people than we think who are environmentally concerned have had transcendent moments of awe in nature that seem best expressed as a feeling of love.[2] That this psychological foundation for nature kinship is not better known and appreciated seems due more to the social reluctance to reveal such experiences than to the lack of people having them. It seems that nature transcendence is a little like sex before the Kinsey reports:

Lots of people are having the experiences, but few are bold enough to talk about them publicly or to admit their importance in regard to lifelong attitudes and values.

The root of the word *conservation* and the birth of the modern conservation movement can be traced to just such a mystical experience that took place at a special place in nature. Gifford Pinchot, chief forester in the administration of President Theodore Roosevelt, knew the outdoors well as a sportsman, but his special expertise was scientific forestry. Roosevelt asked Pinchot to come up with a single unitive policy directive that could be employed to guide resource management for a wide range of environmental issues, including fisheries, wildlife, forestry, public lands, mining, mineral leasing, oil drilling, parklands, and so on. Pinchot found the magnitude and complexity of this assignment overwhelming, so, on a foggy February morning in 1905, he slowly rode his horse, named Jim, through Rock Creek Park in Washington, D.C., deeply depressed. Suddenly, surrounded by the splendor of the ravine, he recalled that in India there were large districts called conservancies, which the government managed for the good of everyone. This insight, he reports in his autobiography, was like a flash of light at the end of a long tunnel. The words "the greatest good for the greatest number for the longest time" came to mind, and he dug his spurs into Jim and raced back to the White House with his revelation, rushing into Roosevelt's office to tell him the news. Roosevelt became excited and called a special cabinet meeting that evening, during which Secretary McGee coined the word *conservation* to describe the new guiding policy of the Roosevelt administration: "The wise use of natural resources for the greatest number of people for the longest time."[3] It was not that Pinchot was unconcerned before this moment of ecstatic insight, but that the noetic quality of the truth revealed in that moment became an inspiration that moved his own ecological action to a higher level, as well as that of millions of others for generations to come.

A recent U.S. government study has shown that the average

adult today in the United States spends 84 percent of his or her life indoors. Much of this time is spent in environments with artifically controlled temperature, light, humidity, and air circulation. And while we're enclosed by four walls, reality becomes determined more and more by forces other than our own perceptual awareness; television commentators become our new eyes, ears, and noses. Reading the cloud patterns in the sky to forecast the weather is now turned over to the weatherman and his satellite photos. The songs of birds, whales, and wolves are heard on cassettes; seldom do we thrill to the real thing. Reality becomes more and more secondhand. Some say that Socrates is responsible for our retreat from nature, for he declared that nothing of importance took place outside the walls of the city. In all fairness to the urbane Greek philosopher (who ultimately had to face his antinature karma by drinking a lethal herbal potion of hemlock), two potent forces of modern cultural conditioning are more guilty of pulling people away from nature:

The first is a modern religious system that dismisses nature worship as being synonymous with the devil and has turned religion into a process of building community to support the church rather than the full range of human spiritual needs. By and large, churches have failed to provide ways for people to achieve deeply personal experiences of spirituality that enable them to fully realize human existence and their capacity to individuate. Religious services and readings point people's attention to the afterlife and to a God in the sky, but neglect the fact that churches are sited on tracts of land that influence the spirituality of what takes place there, and that the rich early traditions of all great religions acknowledge that God is unveiled through communion with nature at special places.

The second force is a Newtonian-Cartesian scientific mechanical paradigm that says that all things can be explained by physics and chemistry and measured by external objective standards. When we allow schedules, slide rules, calculus, clocks, and machines to guide our life's direction and purpose, instead of the subtle pull of the cycling of the sun, the moon, the tides, the seasons, and our holistic intuitive perception, we deny ourselves the chance to participate in reality fully. When we allow our children's schools to be organized according to mechanical schedules and their success to be determined in achievement-test scores rather than self-worth, self-awareness, and health of the children, we are telling children they should learn to be machines, not people. When people believe they are no longer as important as machines, then soul is set aside in favor of regularity, and creativity dwindles into routine acts carried out by production lines, rather than creating self-fulfilling craftsmanship. Drug abuse, alcoholism, anxiety, hypochondria, and escapist pursuits become common in an attempt to compensate for that part of life that machines have gobbled up and hidden away from our perception.

If we maintain that each place doesn't have its own unique spirit, presence, and power, we are living a lie. When we assert that we do not and cannot communicate with nature and gain wisdom, we have lost the root of spirituality. Deny our sensory linkages to nature and we become seduced by whims and fantasies to distract us from acknowledging our feelings of quiet desperation.

Several years ago I participated in a national task force on water-resources management sponsored by the U.S. Army Corps of Engineers. One proposal that arose from think-tanking with Pentagon brass was periodically using the media to create environmental disasters, just to keep people aware of the ecology, in much the same fashion that we have air-raid drills during wartime. The fundraising letters of many environmental groups that almost daily bring news of shocking new disasters and appeals for funding have probably stopped the Pentagon's scheme with overkill.

We think and create as a reflection of who we are inside. Problems in the world around us indicate inner conflicts and voids as much as faulty calculations. We have lost that primal kinship link with nature that shamans and modern psychological research both agree is the key to living a vital, full, and creative life. We continue to act in ways that disrupt the ecology because our thinking is pulled away from knowing how to turn inward and our senses are dulled in looking outward to receive guidance from the subtle rhythms and symbols that want to guide us into a symphony in celebration of wholeness. Environmental problems will be solved and prevented when people can change their inner lives to regain the primal linkage with nature that is the root of healthy action. It will require getting up out of the armchair, discovering our senses, and learning to trust voices and feelings we have been led to believe were not there.

THE POWER OF A SPECIAL PLACE

Out at Point Reyes National Seashore, located just north of San Francisco, there is a restored Coastal Miwok Indian village named Kule Loklo. In the middle of a clearing ringed by stately eucalyptus trees a pronounced mound emerges from the earth like a primordial turtle. Upon closer inspection, the mound is the ceiling of an underground ceremonial dance house called a *lamma.*

The Coastal Miwok who once lived here are long gone, victims of disease and the new religion, but today the keepers of Kule Loklo are two very special National Park Service employees, Lanny and Esther Pinola, both Kashaya Pomo Indians with some bloodlines tracing back to the Coastal Miwok people. You have to stoop down to enter the passageway, like squeezing down a birth canal of the second mother, the earth. Inside her womb you can again stand in a room some nine to ten feet tall, supported by twelve bay-tree trunks around the perimeter, with four sturdy columns of giant bay trees closer to the center, one for each of the directions: north, west, south, and east. In the middle there is a massive center pole made from a grandfather bay's trunk, blackened on one side from ceremonial fires lit in a pit directly under the smoke hole in the ceiling.

There is a special feeling in this place. The air, which is scented by the sweet odors of bay leaves burned in many ritual fires, seems especially light and charged with softness. "There is much *weya* here," says Esther quietly. *Weya* in Pomo means "spirit." Not long ago this *lamma* was open all the time, but today there is a lock on the wooden door at the entrance. The restricted access is due to two forces: One is vandalism, some of which is apparently racial; and the other is the popularity of the space, which requires almost constant supervision because so many people feel drawn to it.

"Not long ago we found a woman in here, shaking and shivering," Lanny says quietly. "We thought she was sick, but it turned out that she was a nun who felt drawn to this place as if by a magnetic force. In the rain she came out and sat down inside the *lamma* and felt overwhelmed by the experience of being there, for, in her own words, 'For the first time in my life I was in a real church.' "

Lanny and Esther have so often found themselves called to be counselors for people like this woman who feel called to the spirit of Kule Loklo. "They are remembering," Lanny says simply, "remembering who they are, why they are here, and what the spirit is."

In the forthcoming pages of this book we will undertake a journey in search of the primal wilderness of the human mind and its potential to form intimate kinship relationships with the energies, forces, creatures, and even spirits of nature. This trek will take us through two relatively untraveled territories—shamanistic psychology and the cutting edge of modern consciousness research—and offer a practical synthesis to enable you to benefit more fully from having the powers of nature alive and at work in your life.

Whereas we moderns stumble into experiences of nature kinship and lack a psychology to comprehend them, traditional peoples plan for them with elaborate ceremonies and rituals, drawing upon a knowledge of environmental psychology that far surpasses that conjured up by modern psychology. While modern people dig for the yellow metal gold, which the Sioux call *maza zi,* the real precious gold we need sparkles in the eyes of elders, the clear essence of being human, at peace with nature and self, living the memory of being descended from tens of thousands of years of human evolution. Fortunately more and more people are recognizing that there is this priceless treasure there, just as so many tribes are on the verge of extinction.

The other great source of help we can consult in our search for nature kinship is humanistic and transpersonal psychology. The lessons of Gestalt therapy developed by Fritz Perls taught us that we create as an expression of who we are inside. Gobbling up electrical energy and natural resources and using chemicals to satisfy every whim—this is the mirror image of the insecurity that drives us to achieve, consume for status and anxiety, and ingest chemical stimulants and sedatives to control our moods. One of the first to call attention to the connection between burnout within and burnout around us was the Swedish economist Staffan B. Linder, who in 1970 published an insightful and troubling study entitled "The Harried Leisure Class," in which he showed how when people embrace an ever-growing gross national product as their primary social goal, life becomes more and more hectic and less and less fulfilling. One result of this pattern is that "people die an early death from overstrain and insufficient time instead of, as previously, from a shortage of goods. Deaths are now caused by high productivity, not low productivity."[4] In one of the greatest insights into the ecological dilemma of our times, Fritz Perls proclaimed, "We do to ourselves as we do the environment."

Abraham Maslow added to Perls's wisdom when, after years of studying the depths of the human psyche, he declared, "Not only is man PART of nature, and it part of him, but also he must be at least minimally isomorphic with nature (similar to it) in order to be viable in it. It has evolved him. His communion with what transcends him therefore need not be defined as nonnatural or supernatural. It may be seen as 'biological experience.' "[5]

More and more people are agreeing that we have to regain a sense of harmony with nature. Few, however, understand the territory of the soul we'll have to recover. The shelves of bookstores today are filled with self-help guides to help you turn inward and take more responsibility for your life and health. Beside them are scores of helpful guides to help you develop more enriching relationships with other people and increase sexual pleasure. On another shelf you find volumes of nature and ecology books. Some describe natural history with beautiful photos of birds, flowers, animals, and scenery. Still others probe environmental problems and offer economic, political, and personal solutions for conserving resources and cleaning up the earth. Strangely enough, next to nothing describes how to develop better psychological health through more intimate contact with the natural world. If we lived in a traditional society, most self-help books would stress techniques for recovering nature kinship. Can it be that by becoming civilized we no longer have the same psychic root as traditional cultures? Such an evolutionary change in so short a time would be the equivalent of growing wings.

This book offers a psychology of nature kinship that arises from my experiences as a naturalist, counselor, researcher, and companion of native peoples over nearly three decades. It is a map of the wilderness of the mind and some suggestions for befriending this domain so that you too can feel what Chief Joseph of the Nez Percé meant when he said, "The earth and I are of one mind." This is a guidebook of practical wizardry.

Nature

as Teacher

and Healer

Chapter One

RETURNING TO
THE ROOTS

*If every individual had
a better relation to the
animal within him, he would
also set a higher value on life.*

—CARL GUSTAV JUNG
Civilization in Transition

Among many tribal cultures the place where a person was born and raised provides an important description of his or her identity and power—a kind of charm, you might say. I was born and raised on Grosse Ile, Michigan, an island in Lake Erie at the mouth of the Detroit River. While many kids earn their first spending money with a paper route, I earned my first pocket cash trapping muskrats, helping commercial fishermen unload their catch, guiding my father's friends for duck hunting and perch fishing on Lake Erie, and carrying filled gallon jugs of mineral water to people's cars, for my family owns a large, flowing artesian well, which you'll hear more about later. I'm an only child, and for me my brothers and sisters have always been ducks, fish, trees, cattail marshes, and the wind.

There's a power of place that we've forgotten about. The Greeks spoke of the *genius loci,* or the "spirit" of place, and sited the temple to honor Gaia, the earth goddess, at Delphi, as they felt it favored her work of moving human minds to prophesy. Astrologers insist that each place is uniquely aligned with the heavens, forever influencing the lives of those born there. Another more recent theory about the power of place says that as you're being formed in your mother's womb, the unique energies of the place where your mother was during the later stages of pregnancy leave a special imprint in the molecular structure of your forming bones, which will be there for the rest of your life. When two or more objects vibrate at the same frequency, harmony is achieved and energy is exchanged. Thus, forever after you're harmonically linked with the place of your birth in a manner that energizes your life regardless of where you are on the surface of the earth, like being plugged into an invisible electric power plant.[1]

In psychoanalysis they say that your earliest memories often have a profound influence on your later psychological development. Two early vivid memories stand out in my mind as being harbingers of my interest in ecology. One November afternoon when I was six or seven years old, my father took me out duck hunting with him for the first time. We crouched in an old blind with a frame of woven willows covered with golden cattails as the west wind swept by in great gusts, making the rushes sound like rattles of invisible spirit dancers, while out in the lake the white-capped waves leaped high in the air with a passion as swirls of snowflakes sprinkled the crests. There was a snowstorm to the northeast, which was pushing flocks of ducks from Ontario and northern Michigan southward. The churning gray surface of Lake Erie wasn't the kind of place a wing-weary duck would want to settle down onto for the night, so out of that black cloud came flock after flock of exhausted red-legged black ducks with silvery-white underwings sparkling in the late-afternoon sun, seeking shelter from the storm. My father had his limit in minutes, but we just sat there until dark, watching clusters of ducks come tumbling down out of the skies to splash down into the shallow marsh for rest and food. Even now as I recall that memory of some forty years ago, I feel swept back into a timeless zone of human experience that has stirred the deepest parts of the human soul for thousands of years.

About the same time I caught my first fish, a bright little saucer-sized pumpkinseed sunfish that I pounced on once my bamboo pole had carried it from the water to the bank. With ceremony we cleaned and cooked my first catch that night. I was filled with great pride as I took my first bite, only to spit it out immediately with revulsion. "Got a bone in it?" my father asked.

"No," I replied, "but it tastes like oil." He took a bite and also spit it out.

"Too bad," he said, "never used to taste that way in the old days. It's because of the things they dump in the river."

At an average rate of 175,000 cubic feet per second, the Detroit River surges through a strait less than a mile wide for thirty-one miles, past more than five million people and the automobile-manufacturing capital of the world. As it's swallowed by the shallow basin of Lake Erie, the Great Lake the Huron Indians say has the spirit of a panther, the gray-green fertile waters slip past two cigar-shaped islands, reminiscent of a track of the giant mythic moose Gluskap. Along the Canadian shore lies Bob-Lo, an amusement park. Its more docile twin to the west in American waters is Grosse Ile, today the quiet home of more than twelve thousand people, but once seriously considered as a site for the United Nations, suggesting a sense of its potential as a place of power.

Dr. Noel J. Browne, director of the United Nations Environment Programme, has said, "Incredible transformations and attitude formations await our collective attention and participation in a global effort to restore, protect, and enhance the earth." A history of the Detroit River's use by modern culture reveals many elements of the universal story of how becoming "civilized" has brought about the progressive destruction of natural ecosystems and species. First the French used the Detroit River as a sewer. Each winter in the early 1700s the hay, straw, and manure from all the stables in Detroit would be hauled out onto the frozen river and dumped on the ice so that the spring thaws would carry it away downstream. As Detroit grew from a trading post into a city, the dumping increased. The records for the Detroit City Council for 1823 read, "Mr. Peter Berthelet was authorized to build a wharf from the shore out to deep water and to install a pump to supply water that would be 'free from contamination by the debris commonly dumped into the river.' "

By 1909 the pollution of the Detroit River had grown so bad that an International Joint Commission of representatives from the United States and Canada was formed to look into the problem. They reported four years later that the problem did exist and was the result of both sides dumping untreated sewage into the river. Both sides acknowledged the problem and its sources, and an agreement was reached to build some sewage-treatment plants. A 1929–30 follow-up study concluded that the river was no longer polluted to a harmful degree. My father, who was born on Grosse Ile in 1901 and has lived there nearly all his life, confirms this, recalling how he and his friends used to be able to see the bottom of the river before you dove off the bridge on the west shore.

The treatment of domestic wastes gave the river a temporary reprieve, but as Henry Ford's assembly line grew along with the steel mills and electric power plants that allowed him to create the automobile-manufacturing capital of the world, the river's health declined. Situated halfway between the iron-ore deposits of the Mesabi Range in Minnesota and northern Michigan, and the coalfields of Appalachia, with abundant water for transportation and manufacturing, and sitting on top of massive deposits of limestone to help the blast furnaces turn iron into steel, Detroit was the ideal place to make cars. Fueled by World War II, our growing love affair with the car, and the steady flow of new workers—including Poles, Greeks, Hungarians, blacks, and Appalachian hillbillies—and their families coming to Detroit hoping to jump from poverty into middle-class luxury, industrial pollution and domestic sewage flowed into the river worse than ever when I caught my fateful sunfish. A 1946–48 International Joint Commission examination of the Detroit River reported that it was seriously polluted by some 1,739,120,040 gallons of municipal and industrial waste waters that were flushed away on an average day. Once-abundant species, such as whitefish, blue pike, and sturgeon, had virtually disappeared from Lake Erie before I was born in 1943.

The river was dying, but most people seemed unconcerned, in part because there was no clear and present danger. In earlier times typhoid fever had sometimes swept through the Detroit area due to sewage-laced drinking water, but with chlorination, no one was dying from water pollution in the 1940s. Major public-access sites and bridges displayed big signs warning people that the river was a health hazard. You could still catch fish from the bank, but not the same rich assortment of species you could have landed a few decades before. But new generations moved into the area, not knowing what it was like to have clean water, and older established families now owned boats to catch "clean" fish farther out in the lake. Better still, people bought cabins in northern Michigan that could be reached in just a few short hours thanks to the new highway system. The economy prospered, and with little or no protest, the Detroit River became a national sacrifice in the name of economic growth and employment.

A 1964 International Joint Commission report delivered the bad news. According to this study the lower twenty-six miles of the Detroit River were now "polluted bacteriologically, chemically, physically, and biologically so as to interfere with municipal water supplies, recreation, fish and wildlife propagation and navigation."[2] The water was so bad then that everyone knew this, but almost no one was willing to do anything about it.

Oil spills, such as the 1989 Alaskan spill in Prince William Sound and the massive discharge into the Persian Gulf during the 1991 war over Kuwait, have caught people's attention recently. Growing up on Grosse Ile, it was common to wake up and find a black line of greasy oil along the sides of your boat, evidence the night before, just a few miles up river, a supervisor had decided to open the floodgates of his plant to avoid the costs of treating industrial wastes, letting the quiet surge of the current carry the oil away before dawn. Game biologist Dr. George Hunt, one of my early mentors, estimated that as many as ten thousand swans, ducks, and geese used to die every winter in the lower Detroit River as night migrational flights would alight into oil slicks drifting down the river. The worst damage occurred when the river froze over, because the areas of open water remaining were where waste waters were discharged from the big plants. Already weakened by cold temperatures, the birds would plop down into the warm effluents and be quickly coated with oil. The oil would weigh them down, compact their feathers so that the normal buoyancy and insulation of their plumage would decrease, and as they tried to get rid of the oil by preening their feathers, they ingested the oil, which poisoned them. We grow sick at the sight of oil-soaked birds flopping around on the beach, such as the television news programs show us, but those highly visible birds are a small minority of the total casualties of any spill. Many, many others simply become weak and sink quietly out of sight to the bottom, never to be counted.

Industrialization has also changed the air we breathe. As a child I remember how the steel plants across the river would purge their blast furnaces at night and belch tons of iron-ore particulate matter into the black night sky so that no one could identify the source of the orange snow that greeted us the next morning. Other times clouds of strange fumes would be carried on the west wind, sometimes causing one's eyes to water. An air-quality study of the Detroit-Windsor airshed by the International Joint Commission in the 1960s showed that on the north end of Grosse Ile (where I first lived) the average dustfall per square mile per month was approximately one hundred tons. I suffered from chronic bronchitis, like a lot of downriver people, until I was twelve, when we moved to the southern tip of the island. Despite the damage to property and health, few people protested. A number of people living along the river painted their houses brick red or salmon so that the reddish orange dust couldn't be seen.

When the great psychiatrist Carl Gustav Jung traveled to the United States in the early part of the twentieth century, he remarked that "in America there is a discrepancy between conscious and unconscious that is not found in Europe, a tension between an extremely high level of culture and unconscious primitivity."[3] The source of this conflict, Jung asserted, was that the new modern culture had failed to acknowledge the importance of coming into harmony with the place where you live as a fundamental root of peace and health. Without such a rootedness, Jung said, people are likely to be swept in various directions according to the prevailing sentiments of the times, succumbing to fads and whims rather than acting from a grounded, visceral wisdom that grows into one's mind out of the earth, like the native plants of a bioregion.

I hadn't read Carl Jung when I enrolled in the University of Michigan School of Natural Resources in 1961, but the driving forces of love for nature and hatred of pollution motivated me to want to do something to stop the destruction of the area where I grew up. I began as a Wildlife Management major, further developing the awareness and understanding of nature that I had cultivated since early childhood. I soon decided, however, that the source of environmental problems ultimately lay with people, so I changed my major to conservation education and planned to become a conservation educator.

I loved being outside leading nature hikes. It allowed me to share some of the nature lore I had acquired since childhood, as well as the new concepts I'd learned while getting a bachelor's degree. Being a naturalist also enabled me to be an entertainer with a captive audience.

In two years' time I had become director of the Ann Arbor

schools' K–12 conservation and outdoor education program, which continues to provide field trips for over 90 percent of the elementary school kids in the Ann Arbor system each year. The kids loved the program, and it won several national awards, but I felt it wasn't doing enough about the serious environmental problems in southeastern Michigan. I began a master's degree in water-resources planning and designed a thesis research program to study the economic consequences of water pollution in the lower Detroit River. I wanted to dramatize the problem and mobilize people to clean up the river.

I was quickly able to document millions of dollars of direct and indirect costs to health, drinking-water supplies, recreation, and fish and wildlife. But no one wanted to say anything publicly about the problem. The Detroit Chamber of Commerce slide show of the Rouge River, which flows into the Detroit River just south of downtown Detroit, featured an aerial shot of the Ford Rouge plant going full tilt—to promote new business growth in the area. From the tall stacks of a power plant clouds of black smoke billowed while the muddy-orange oxygen-depleted waters of the Rouge slipped by to stain the Detroit River just a mile or two away. Nearby a red plume laden with particulates erupted from a steel mill. And the Ford Rouge plant labored away with dense clouds of white and black smoke, indicating all shifts working away. Here was an example of the worst air and water pollution in America at that time. Instead the chamber of commerce script called it, proudly, "Detroit, the industrial capital of the Midwest." Today people wonder if the Rouge River got its name from its present state as a reddish-colored flowing dump. No. The French explorers named it for the beautiful red maple trees that once lined its banks.

Not far downstream from where the Rouge River flows into the Detroit, I interviewed a longtime area resident owner of a boat livery. His records showed that right after World War II business had been great, but since then revenues had steadily declined, despite an unprecedented nationwide outdoor recreation boom. As we sat on his dock, talking about his decades along the river, a bright slick of oil washed past with a dead fish in the middle. I asked him why he thought his business was going under. There were two primary reasons, he said. First, everyone had gotten rich in the auto plants and now owned cabins in northern Michigan, where the fishing was better. Of course one of the reasons everyone went north was that the local river was so badly polluted. Second, he said, "The weather's changin'. People just don't go out boating when the weather is bad a lot." If his declining revenues were any indication of weather trends, we would be in an ice age. When asked directly about the quality of water in the river, he just shook his head and started talking about the rising price of worms.

Environmental Psychology

For decades the conventional wisdom of conservation education was to attack problems such as pollution through education by churning out and disseminating tons of educational materials. In all my courses in natural resources, never once was psychology used to explain environmental issues. This seemed strange to me, since all environmental problems arise from human action or nonaction. Fortunately for me, the University of Michigan Graduate School allows joint doctoral programs, so I developed one combining natural resources and psychology and quickly became the focus of many "Paul Bunyan" jokes from the regular psychology students in my new classes.

While nothing was said directly about ecology and pollution in the psychology texts, I found there was a good deal of information that applied to environmental problems. Aristotle was one of the first environmental psychologists in Western thinking. He believed there were three components to the human soul: the "nutritive soul," which is shared with the plant kingdom; the "sensitive soul," which is shared with the animal kingdom; and the "intellectual (or rational) soul," which is solely the property of humans. Like his mentor, Plato, and like Pliny the Elder, the greatest Greek naturalist, Aristotle understood that our minds had many links to nature that, if acknowledged, would result in a natural intuitive understanding of the flows, cycles, systems, and creatures of the natural world.

The connection between science and spirituality was banished by the Renaissance, leaving us with the Newtonian-Cartesian mechanical model of reality, which champions rational objectivity instead of sympathetic intuitive understanding of nature and spirit. The rise of Christianity, with its emphasis on "the word of God" being the Bible rather than the direct experience of God, separated us farther from nature kinship. People like to quote Genesis 1:28 as an indication of Christianity's attitude toward nature: "Be fruitful and multiply, and fill the earth and subdue it; and have dominion over the fish of the sea, over the birds of the air, and over every living thing that moves upon the earth."

If one actually followed this advice and understood ecology, it could lead to a kind of benevolent-stewardship philosophy. In psychology I learned that people's underlying emotional qualities are often more important than their words and are often crucial to understanding human behavior. If you really want to see where Christian dogma makes a fundamental error in ecological thinking, look at the attitude expressed in Genesis 9: 2–3: "The fear of you and the dread of you shall be upon every beast of the earth; and upon every fowl of the air, and upon all that moveth on the earth, and upon all the fishes of the sea." When I recognized the psychological interpretation of this biblical teaching, I understood why some of the worst poachers in the area where I had grown up were also regular churchgoers. Taking this passage from Genesis at face value, you can terrorize fish, deer, and ducks and still be on the right side of Jesus, so long as you love your fellow man.

The Psychology of Change

Studying attitude formation and change, psychologist Herbert Kelman found that people's attitudes are influenced in three general ways:[4]

"Compliance" implies change when faced with an external authority figure, possibly one who uses a threat or an implied threat to make people behave in a certain way. This is the mechanism of law, and it works reasonably well. People will, however, comply with situations they don't believe in out of fear. When this is the case, rebellion is always lurking in the unconscious, waiting for an opportunity to explode into confrontation.

"Identification" implies change inspired by someone a person respects. This is why advertisers use celebrities to sell products, and heroes and heroines can sway public opinion. Success here depends more on charisma and appeal to emotion than on fact, and the success of advertising in influencing consumer behavior is one indication why a rational-empirical approach to nature education has limited effectiveness.

"Internalization" is the most potent type of attitude change or formation process. When you develop an attitude that is consistent with everything inside of you right down to your core, it's the kind of thing that will move you to stand up for what you believe in, even in the face of great opposition. The problem we face today is that many people don't know who or what they are, let alone have an intimate relationship with nature. We sacrifice self-awareness in favor of mastering mental techniques and pay a high price inside and in the world around us. One of the wisest psychological insights on the human condition is that of Jungian analyst Aniela Jaffé, who suggests, "Suppressed and wounded instincts are the dangers threatening civilized man; uninhibited drives are the dangers threatening primitive man."[5]

COMING TO OUR SENSES

One of the biggest criticisms of the modern environmental movement is that it is run almost entirely by middle- and upper-middle-class white people. You get perspective on yourself by looking at how other people experience the world, one professor told me. So, for my doctoral-thesis research I went to Mackenzie High School in Detroit, which is primarily black and in the vicinity of the Ford Rouge plant, where monthly dustfalls averaged 120 tons per square mile. I conducted surveys and interviewed over two hundred high school kids in this area, asking them what they thought about air pollution in their neighborhood.

The kids agreed the air was bad, but many of them had never traveled far beyond their immediate area, so to them the idea of blue sky and fresh air was foreign. "Besides, it don't kill you and you gotta have money to eat," one student said when asked if he'd ever done anything about the conditions where he lived, summing up the overwhelming sentiments of the group. Drugs, crime, and unemployment were the major issues for them. Survival.

The single most important factor in determining serious concern for air pollution among these kids was how frequently they got out of the city and personally experienced clean air and blue skies. There was no significant statistical correlation between how much they knew about air pollution and their desire to do anything about it. This finding, which is supported by research on public opinion on other social issues, underscores the fact that extensive media coverage of ecological problems by itself will not guarantee citizen action and support for pollution control.

I was so moved by the kids I interviewed that I got a grant from the U.S. Department of Health, Education and Welfare to set up a special school for training social activists. The school took place every afternoon after regular school hours five days a week. We ran the program in cooperation with the Urban League, and we brought in Saul Alinsky–trained activists to give the students skills of organizing and problem solving. During the time the free school lasted, the kids created a park for little kids and set up a special job-counseling program for dropouts. When the government funding ran out, we asked the local school board to pick it up, but they rejected it, fearing riots in the schools. The 12th Street Academy died after one year. One of the students went on to get a master's from Berkeley, and I accepted an offer to join the University of Michigan faculty.

A year later David Lingwood, a fellow faculty member at the university, and I trained over one hundred students to administer a questionnaire about air quality in the three Downriver Detroit communities closest to the Ford Rouge plant: Wyandotte, River Rouge, and Ecorse. The UAW and the T.B. and Health Society asked us to conduct the study, and short-haired union workers drove the long-haired students around to gather the data from over five hundred homes. We found that common respiratory diseases and heart disease were as much as eight times the national average in these areas. Nearly everyone reported air-pollution damage to their homes, cars, and gardens. Almost no one had ever complained, however, unless there was a clear and present unbearable situation. Heavy smog was a normal thing. As one person said, "You kind of forget how bad it is when there are so many other immediate things coming down." No one wanted to rock the boat and lose his or her job. People adapted for survival reasons.

Releasing our statistics caused an uproar in the Downriver Detroit area. There were shake-ups in the Detroit Public Health Department and in the city council of Ecorse not long afterward. At public meetings in the area people began to speak up, saying they'd lived there so long that they'd come to accept the smog and dirt in the air and had lost perspective on its harmful effects. Slowly steps were taken to clean up the air.

Studies like these moved Pulitzer Prize–winning scientist

René Dubos, in his book *Man Adapting,* to predict that if we don't blow ourselves up with a nuclear war, the greatest long-term threat to humanity will be from a gradual erosion of the quality of life. Dubos likened our situation to that of a frog jumping into a pot of water that is being heated on a stove. If the rise in temperature is gentle, the frog could swim along merrily, enjoying the warmer water, until eventually he is cooked. This observation underscores the importance of preserving wild places so that we have a baseline for people to understand what environmental quality really means.

This research represented pioneering work in environmental psychology. When I spoke at the first national conference on environmental education in the spring of 1970 in Green Bay, Wisconsin, it was the first time anyone could recall that environmental education had been linked with psychological concepts such as attitudes and values. When I published my research, I was deluged with offers to make speeches. I received numerous awards and was invited to consult with public-interest groups, national associations, businesses, and a White House Conference. In the spring of 1970 I appeared at twenty-two Earth Day teach-ins around the United States as a speaker and musician and was part of the central planning committee for the nation's largest college eco-teach-in, held at the University of Michigan.

The university ENACT teach-in drew fifty thousand people. One of the keynote speakers was ecologist Barry Commoner. After Commoner had finished speaking to a capacity crowd of twelve thousand enthusiastic people, he and I found ourselves alone together in a room backstage. We talked about a variety of things, and then Barry went silent and stared into space for a minute with a look of awe on his face. When he again looked at me, he looked me in the eye and said with great seriousness, "You know tonight we've started something so powerful that none of us can really know now how profound a change this is going to have on society. It's going to spread everywhere—politics, education, health care, even religion." How true his prophecy has become!

Chapter Two

LEARNING TO
SURRENDER

*The earth is real, and we are obliged
by the fact of our utter dependence
on it to listen more closely
to its messages.*
—WILLIAM RUCKELSHAUS
"Toward a More Sustainable World,"
Scientific American

In Chinese philosophy it is said that unknown seeds of change
are found in every pinnacle of success. Not long after Earth Day
my marriage broke up, and the resulting emotional pain was
strong enough that I felt a need to retreat inside myself. I got into
psychoanalysis and there learned from my analyst one of the
most important lessons of psychology. Lying on his couch, I gave
a lecture on myself in psychological terms based on what I'd
read. He listened patiently and then quoted Carl Jung, "No
textbook can teach psychology: one learns only by actual experience."

These words shot through me like a bullet. In a few weeks I
moved to a small undeveloped lake outside of Ann Arbor and got
rid of my television set. Good therapy lubricates your dreams as
it releases the lid on the unconscious. One of my analyst's early
comments was how angry I was. Not long after I moved to the
lake, a vivid dream one night showed the right side of my head
swelling up as if it were going to explode. In analysis I learned
this indicated repression of my feminine side. This became

clearer when I learned that of the four functions of consciousness that Jung identified—thinking, feeling, sensation, and intuition—my dominant mode of being was intuition.

As a result of self-confrontation in eight months of analysis, I stopped writing, realizing that my emotions colored my ability to think clearly, and vowed not to resume until I had something fresh to say that wasn't colored by my own inner process. A few months later I turned down a job opportunity with the Smithsonian Institution and moved to tiny Bellingham, Washington, to begin teaching at a small, new environmental-studies program at Huxley College. I set three goals for myself: continue self-exploration, seek to understand the roots of love for nature, spend more time enjoying life.

The process of coming to terms with one's own inner self often begins with an unexpected calling that may come in strange ways, as if nature is inviting you to make a personal transformation. In the backwoods of New England the old-timers say that important upcoming events can be foretold. They are revealed by "forerunners," which include dreams, animal behavior, moods of weather, children's play, and unusual events. To get deeper into myself, I began taking sessions in Reichian breathing, a deep therapy that seeks to unlock chronic muscle tension through hyperventilation and massage. In one session I hyperventilated into a state called apnea, a loss of consciousness due to excessive oxygen, and slipped into a velvetlike inky-black world. A tunnel opened up, and I found myself slipping downward. Popping out of this tube, I found myself in a skin hut, surrounded by Eskimos! We went outside, got into a boat, and went out whaling. Suddenly the boat began to rise from the ocean. Looking down, I saw we were on top of a giant sperm whale. The whale looked up at me, opened his mouth, and I went down into his gaping gullet. I began to hear a snapping sound, which I thought was my bones being crunched by the whale, but instead I discovered it was my therapist snapping his fingers and clapping to wake me up. The whole experience was like being thrust into the most vivid dream you can imagine, and my therapist did not want to talk about it!

Back at Huxley a new student appeared in my classes. He was deeply tanned and had a wild look in his eyes. He reported to the class that he had just hiked the entire length of the proposed trans-Alaskan pipeline, and fascinated us with tales of wolves, bears, eagles, caribou, and glaciers. After class he told me if I ever wanted to go to Prudhoe Bay to see the Alaskan oilfields before the pipeline went in, he could get me from Anchorage to Prudhoe Bay for free.

I thanked him, but I really had not been thinking of going to Alaska. Instead I was preoccupied by an invitation from the Sierra Club to make a speech at their national convention. They wanted me to talk about improving their public relations, and they suggested it would be useful to do this with a specific case study. A nuclear power plant had been proposed for the nearby Skagit Flats in Washington, so I tried to organize a group of students to help me survey people in the area where the plant would be built. I made announcements in all the classes that I was looking for people to do work on this survey, but no one volunteered. I was disappointed. Then out of the blue came a job offer at the University of Oregon from one of my former thesis advisers at the University of Michigan. I called Jim Kelly in Oregon, and he described the job, adding that he would include some money for research "for something like studying what people think about the Alaskan pipeline that's about to go in."

First the apnea experience. Then the student. Then Kelly's offer of money. I didn't know then that strong omens often come in threes, but I sensed something unusual was going on. I accepted the offer from the University of Oregon and began planning a summer trip to Alaska.

That summer I walked, drove, and flew the entire route of the proposed Alaskan pipeline from Prudhoe Bay on the Arctic Ocean to Valdez and out to Kodiak Island, interviewing everyone I could, especially people with bumper stickers like SIERRA KISS MY AXE, SIERRA GO HOME, and LET THE BASTARDS FREEZE IN THE DARK. One day at the end of the trip I walked out of my hotel in Anchorage and found a group of Eskimos in the parking lot. They had just come in from King Island out in the Bering Sea to raise money for a medical clinic. They proposed to do this by doing public performances. I was enchanted by their songs and dances, but few people noticed them, since the Eskimos knew nothing about getting media attention. I volunteered to help with some calls to the *Anchorage Daily News* and local radio and television stations. Within a few hours they were famous, and crowds began to gather.

A couple of days later, as they were doing their last dance, they asked me to join them. I was captivated by the warmth, energy, and gentleness of these short people, and I quickly joined in their dancing and singing. Their entire band seemed like a giant, loving, happy colonial organism reaching out to engulf me. As we danced, I felt a strange softness slip into me, and it seemed as though everything slowed down. Soft halos of light appeared around people, and I recalled that I had known such a state once or twice playing football in high school and college. The leader of the group looked at me, and it seemed that a spark of light jumped between his eyes and mine and flowed gently all the way down to the bottom of my soul.

A minute or two later they stopped. The leader walked over to me and asked me if I remembered the chanting and dancing steps. I said I did. He then told me that I should go out someplace special and chant and dance, a place like Denali, also known as Mount McKinley. Then they packed up kids, blankets, and drums and left.

Two days later I drove to Denali National Park. As the late-afternoon light was painting the snowcapped summit of Denali golden, I walked along a trail beside a rushing glacial stream. I came to a bluff overlooking a deep hole in the river choked with salmon. Spontaneously I began to chant and dance as the Eskimos had taught me. A sense of excitement washed through me, and I began again to enter that magical slow-motion state of consciousness. Then a strange thing happened. I felt a rush of energy, and a chill went down my spine like a bolt of lightning. I began to shake and tremble. I became terrified and thought I might be dying. In that moment I looked up at the last pink glow of sunlight on Denali's summit and decided that if I was going to die, this was at least a beautiful place to end my life.

I was shaking so hard I had to lie down. For the next half hour I shook and trembled. During this time I felt the presence of the Eskimos around me, and I remembered the apnea experience and the Eskimos in the parking lot in Anchorage in great detail. Then the strange energy slipped away.

Exhausted, I got up and began walking back to camp. A few yards down the trail I turned a corner and came upon an excavation that looked like a grave. A chill rushed down my spine. Then I saw a sign announcing it was an archeological dig. I later found that I had been standing on a place that was probably a route from the earliest Paleolithic land-bridge migrations from Siberia.

Several days later I returned to Eugene, Oregon. Over lunch I told some friends about my experience. As I talked, I could see fear growing in them. Several colleagues in psychology suggested I get a physical to see if I had epilepsy, and left nervously. Only one person remained, an anthropologist who had worked with Indians. "Be careful, don't go back," he said quietly. I asked him what he meant. He replied that sometimes anthropologists who got too close to people they were studying would give up modern life and try to live like them. "Castaneda's gone crazy," he said, and left abruptly.

SUGGESTION: STUDY YOUR PREMONITIONS   Identifying "forerunners" is nearly a lost art, yet we all have feelings about things that are going to happen. When you have an idea that something is going to happen, for whatever reason, write down your prediction. Once a month take out your predictions and look them over. Look for accuracy as well as patterns of interpretation or misinterpretation. This will help you learn to recognize forerunners and also identify some unconscious fears and issues that may be slanting your perceptions of life.

Several weeks later I flew to California for a workshop at the Esalen Institute. I had become friends with Esalen founder Michael Murphy and I related my Denali experience to him. Michael looked at me intently for a few moments, and then with a serious twinkle in his eye he asked me if I knew anything about shamanism. I replied no, I'd never even heard of it. "You'd better start reading," he said. Then he added, "When the call comes, you've got to surrender. It will lead you to where you need to go if you let go and trust that a higher purpose is at work."

Back in Eugene I went to the library and found several books about shamanism, including Mircea Eliade's classic *Shamanism: Archaic Techniques of Ecstasy*. The material was interesting, but as the title indicated, it seemed like something out of the distant past with little relevance to modern life and times.

Several months later, out of the blue, I was approached to join a special team of humanist scholars who were going to help the Klamath and Modoc Indians. In Ann Arbor I had gotten some training in conflict-resolution skills, and soon I found myself negotiating a hot dispute between Indians who had lost their land and some local officials and police. Both sides agreed to check their guns at the door before the meetings began, and things often hovered on the edge of open conflict in the sessions.

During these meetings I became close with an Indian group called the Organization of Forgotten Americans, especially an older Indian woman named Marie Norris. Marie and her son, Fritz, told me old stories of myths and legends and sang traditional songs they were collecting. One day Marie told me that when the Vietnam War began, some Klamaths and Modocs who were drafted went out into the woods alone for several days and prayed. Those who did, she said, all came back alive. I asked what they did, and she gave me some instructions for a wilderness solo according to her traditions.

I had spent a good deal of time alone in nature, so I really didn't think this would be anything special, although my experience in Alaska still lurked in my mind. Soon I went off for three days of fasting in the lava beds of the North Cascades near Mount Bachelor. I took off my clothes, took a short swim in a cold lake, wrapped myself in a blanket, said a prayer, and began a fast. A gentle calmness seemed to pervade all things as darkness fell. Trout dimpled on the surface of the lake, and a pack of coyotes and some owls began a concert.

Every hour or two I said prayers. I had been through quite a bit of therapy at that point, but to my surprise, unexpected emotions began welling up in me. Sitting quietly, my whole life passed through my mind, and I discovered old sources of joy as well as long-suppressed emotional wounds. For the next three days I laughed, cried, and felt cleaner and lighter than ever before. Several times deer walked right up to me and flocks of tiny kinglets landed on my blanket. One night a raccoon crawled over me.

At that time I was living in a cabin in the woods twenty miles north of Eugene near the tiny town of Marcola. As I turned the corner onto the county road that led to the cabin, I suddenly felt a deep sense of sadness and pain. I pulled over to the side of the road to catch my breath. Strange voices seemed to be calling out to me, screaming with terror and anger. I gathered myself together and drove slowly toward my house. As I approached, the feelings grew stronger. Pulling up in front of the house, I was shocked to see that my new next-door neighbor had clear-cut his land while I was gone. I realized in that moment that the pain I had been feeling was the souls of the trees that had been cut, friends I had often sat with in the past. I called a psychic woman

I had met named Olgamaria Galambos, and she advised me to sprinkle cornmeal over the stumps and pray for the spirits of the dead trees. I did, and the voices and feelings of pain subsided.

When I reported this experience to some fellow professors, they just shook their heads. Some fifteen years later physicist Ed Wagner reported in *Northwest Science* magazine that trees communicate with one another by means of W-waves, which travel at about three feet per second through trees and fifteen feet per second through the air. Wagner reports that when one tree is chopped down, it puts out a "tremendous cry of alarm while adjacent trees put out smaller ones." Every mother knows that she can sense her child's emotions. People can feel the same sort of sympathy with places, plants, and animals, especially if they have a special fondness for them, I discovered. Such sensitivity, I've come to see, is a fundamental element in finding true kinship with nature, enabling the mind to engage in meaningful interactions with the tribes and creatures of nature.

In the words of Tatanga Mani, or Walking Buffalo, of the Stoney tribe of Canada, "Did you know that trees can talk? Well, they do. They talk to each other, and they'll talk to you if you listen. Trouble is, white people don't listen. They never learned to listen to the Indians, so I don't suppose they'll listen to the other voices of nature. But I have learned a lot from trees; sometimes about the weather, sometimes about animals, sometimes about the Great Spirit!"[1]

As a result of experiences such as I've briefly described here and others, I began to teach courses on human potentiality. This soon meant I became the "tolerated crazy" on campus. I was the focus of jokes about being a "touchy-feely," but I also was called to help whenever someone on campus freaked out—"because we thought you'd understand them," said one faculty member, who phoned me to help her with a student who had flipped out during final-exam week and thought he was a dog. Soon I had a part-time practice working with people recovering from drug overdoses and other mind-loosening experiences.

About two months after the crying-trees incident I suddenly became ill with a high fever. Some friends called and asked if I needed help. I was about to ask them to take me to the hospital, when Olgamaria called. I respected her because she had once been one of the closest associates of the East Indian swami Paramahansa Yogananda. She told me I was having a "spiritual illness" and that I should stay home, be quiet, and not take any medicine, as the illness would be gone in three days. Somehow I felt a deep truth in her words and I followed her instructions, even though I had a horrible case of nausea and diarrhea. During the next two days I had weird dreams of a family of giant apes who lived inside a magic mountain. Finally, on the morning of the third day, I awoke to find an Indian dressed in bright red colors standing at the foot of my bed. I noticed he was translucent and decided he must be a spirit. The Indian then introduced himself to me as Red Feather and told me he would be a guide for me. I asked him how, and he simply said that he would be with me in my dreams.

A few hours later the fever subsided, and I quickly got well. Not long afterward a friend who was familiar with Carl Jung's work suggested that I read *Civilization in Transition*. When I came to the section entitled "Indianization," I discovered that Jung found that in his therapy with troubled Americans, when they had a dream or vision with an Indian, it usually signaled that a deep healing was taking place, because an earthy sense of self had been accessed. Jung called this the "soul of the Indian" and said that this symbol came to Americans because the Indian symbolized a sense of coming into harmony with the land. Within a year after meeting Red Feather, I got married, resigned from the University of Oregon, and moved to Seattle to set up a private practice as a counselor and create a nonprofit educational organization to sponsor seminars and workshops on health, healing, and spirituality. Red Feather had a strong hand in all this happening, appearing in dreams to remind me to follow my deepest inner voices of rightness, which sometimes came from animals in my dreams.

An important insight into what had been happening to me came one day in a conversation with Dr. Elmer Green of the Menninger Foundation. Listening to my story, Elmer told me of an old Sufi formula for self-development that goes, Align yourself with nature, develop your mind, visualize your future, and act accordingly. The Sufis believe that real learning takes place only when you are in sympathy with the teacher, mind to mind, not with spoken words. If nature is to be the true teacher, you have to get in sympathy with nature so that you can hear the teachings with what the Lummi Indians call the third ear.

Therapy had allowed me to vent pent-up anger and frustration, which helped heal me. As I healed, however, I also lost interest in being an environmental activist. What captured my attention now were the strange experiences that began to unfold in my life. They seemed to make it easy for me to understand the spaces people were going through in both emotional turmoil and spiritual emergence. Inspired by the work of psychiatrist Stanislav Grof on the varieties of spiritual experiences, I began to work more and more as a counselor with people who were making voyages into the wilderness areas of the psyche, and I established a regional center for such people.

From 1977 to 1982 I lived in Seattle, Washington, immersed in a strange caldron of boiling waters of the psyche. By day, as a counselor, I sat and listened to people flipped out on bad trips from chemicals, various personal-growth trainings, overnight-enlightenment seminars, and peak experiences in sports. On evenings and weekends, at the Life Systems Center, which I directed, we had a full program of workshops and seminars which included anthropologist Ashley Montagu, runner Mike Spino, new-age researcher Marilyn Ferguson, naturopath Jack Schwarz, healer Rev. Olga Worrall, and a number of shamans, including Joan Halifax, José Geller, Sun Bear, Prem Das, and

Rolling Thunder. I also helped produce two memorable pro-grams by mythologist Joseph Campbell. Many of these people stayed at our house in the guest room in the basement.

As each passed through, their energies stirred up my psyche, and an extraordinary caravan of dreams began to unfold. Each different type of therapy seems to shape its own unique style of dreaming, I had learned. Analysis seems to encourage compli-cated scenes with many characters, like a Hollywood spectacular. The dreams of Gestalt and Reichian therapy are more immedi-ate, physical, and emotional. Now, however, new forms of dreams began to appear that did not seem to be personal but rather transpersonal. Medicine man Rolling Thunder counseled me one day that there are two types of dreams: dreams of the body, which pertain to personal matters; and dreams of the spirit world. These latter kinds of dreams are very powerful, Rolling Thunder advised, the sort of thing people pray for on mountain-tops. They can drive you crazy if you aren't ready for them.

In shamanic psychology nature is really two interwoven reali-ties: a material plane and a parallel spiritual realm. All around the world shamans assert that the spiritual dimension, where time and space collapse into a unity, is the place from which events in the physical plane originate. This is why shamans strive to master altered states of consciousness, so that they know and influence things before they manifest in this reality.

One of Rolling Thunder's favorite sayings is that if you live your life right, your whole life, twenty-four hours a day, becomes a ritual. At first when he said this, I thought it was a joke. But as the days and weeks passed, my dreams at night were often as bizarre and strange as the experiences of my clients by day, and I had no control over them. There were times when I felt as if I were going crazy. Visiting shamans just laughed and told me that my feeling crazy in this situation was because I had been taught to deny all experiences other than those in temporal, practical reality. I had to hold on to my center and let go of all

other judgments about what reality should be like, they counseled. I finally found a sense of peace when I decided I was myself
a research program in consciousness studies.

One of my first important spirit dreams took place one afternoon when I lay down for a nap following a weekend workshop
on shamanism I produced for Venezuelan psychiatrist José
Geller, who is also an initiated shaman in the Maria Lionza
religion of Venezuela. In this dream it was twilight, and I found
myself lying on a blanket in a forest. From all sides animals
stepped forward, eyeing me. Then a giant raccoon emerged from
the crowd. He licked his lips and proceeded to eat my entire
body while the other animals cheered.

Following this dream I began to have dreams of stones and
crystals that would be placed inside my transparent body. With
each came certain colors, sounds, and images, similar to scenes
from Walt Disney's *Fantasia.* One night I had a singing lesson
in a dream. I looked down at myself and saw I was transparent.
I opened my mouth, and energy came from an area of an inner
organ and formed a mandala in the air in front of me; now I
could see what perfect pitch meant! To my amazement a whole
new range in my voice began to open up.

Once the stones were in place, I began to have a series of
dreams of the taxonomic system of all the plants and animals of
the world, beginning with the simplest microorganisms and
working up to the most complex. One night it would be squid,
shellfish, and octopus. Another night it would be sponges, proto-
zoa, fish, ferns, or trees. They would parade past my eyes as if
I were watching a movie on taxonomic classification. Then at the
end of the dream sequence one would move from the background and be drawn into my body, filling up part of the void
left by the giant raccoon's banquet. Rolling Thunder explained
to me that this is how I was being aligned with nature, so that
I could "think right." I was gathering my kinship allies in nature
through harmonic attraction. During this time I was interviewed
by University of Florida psychiatrist Stanley Dean in a study of

people who have had "ultraconscious experiences." Dean and I concluded that I had had at least ten different kinds of dreams.

Periodically during this time Red Feather would appear in dreams, providing useful information. In one dream he advised me to "study the sacred places, there's something important there." This has resulted in more than a decade of research, which has yielded two books and several symposiums.

I went through "rebodying" in my dreams for two years. It took this long because after each new object entered me, I would need to develop a new integration. As my rebodying came to an end, one day medicine-man Sun Bear asked me if I would like to produce a special event for him based on his dreams. I said I'd be happy to, and Sun Bear said that was good, but first we'd have to ask someone else. I thought he meant he would have to call another medicine man, Mad Bear Anderson, who was a kind of godfather for many Indian medicine people. Sun Bear chuckled and said no, he meant that we would have to ask the Great Spirit by holding a dream ceremony. The modern word *powwow,* he explained, comes from the Algonquin word *pauwaw,* which means "he who dreams."

That night he conducted the ceremony with sixty-five people present, asking for guidance and smoking a medicine pipe that once had belonged to the great Oglala Sioux seer Black Elk. I found myself in a new kind of dream that night, like a Technicolor Steven Spielberg movie of extraordinary clarity. Sun Bear and I walked into a log cabin that was filled with many Indian leaders of the past including Wovoka, who created the Ghost Dance; Sitting Bull; Chief Joseph; and others I did not recognize. They looked us over sternly, and then a door in the back of the cabin opened. I walked out into a clearing ringed by giant trees. I hung a wreath of holly leaves on a wall, and from the woods to the north three giant wooden statues emerged, with massive faces and eyes looking directly at me. I heard the word *manitou* spoken, and I woke up.

Following this dream a series of dreams began that guided me to the location of the First Medicine Wheel Gathering, helped me select speakers, the menu, the program structure, and even how much to charge. In these dreams medicine man Mad Bear Anderson would appear. In physical form Mad Bear looked like the late football coach Woody Hayes, and in these dreams Mad Bear was dressed as a football coach with a clipboard on which he would write directions. As long as I followed his instructions, everything would work out perfectly, and in September 1980 six hundred people attended this event held at the foot of Mount Rainier.

Mixed in the series of dreams about the Medicine Wheel Gathering were a number of dreams with northern Indian symbols. By chance I asked my mother, whose family was from Canada, if we had any Indian blood. She replied that her father was part Indian. I had never met him, for he had died before I was born, but I began to see that by doing acts of service to a higher purpose I would be given unexpected rewards in dreams and other life events.

Not long after the First Medicine Wheel Gathering was completed, I had another extraordinarily vivid dream. The setting for this dream was a fall afternoon on a small island in Lake Erie where I used to hunt and fish. A west wind was blowing up whitecaps, and to the east a flock of white snow geese emerged from a dark snowstorm cloud. The birds flew toward me, and as they began to set their wings to land in the calmer water, they turned into short, dark-skinned, bare-chested men wearing leather pants. The leader of the group landed on the beach carrying a white candle. With a very serious look on his face he walked up to me and shoved the white candle into my chest. I woke up crying.

On Rolling Thunder's advice I then traced the ancestry of my father's side of the family, discovering that the Swans were part of the Gunn Clan of northern Scotland. The Gunns, I found, had come to Scotland from Norway, led by a short, dark-haired king named Olaf the Black. Since most Scandinavians are tall and light, it was clear that Olaf was of Lapp or Saami blood. I then recalled my earlier experiences with the Eskimos in Alaska and realized that I had been dreaming of this branch of my ancestry.

Jung warned Americans that when he said that they should take on the "soul of the Indian," he meant that they should recover their basic harmony with the land where they lived, which in America was symbolized by the form of an Indian. He did not want people to become what Indians call wannabees, people who reject their own roots and imitate Indians. This can lead them to self-delusion, as well as angering Indians, who charge that their culture and religion are being stolen and commercialized.

Modern rational, mechanized society has wrongly guided us away from two of our most important psychic roots—kinship with nature and our ancestral heritage. One result is alienation and anger, for whenever you deny a basic part of yourself, inner hatred begins to build. This inner hatred then gets turned into either psychosomatic illness or aggression or both. Instead of going back, which implies letting go of everything in modern society and living in primitive conditions, we should strive to "extend back" to our roots in nature and in our own ancestry. All of us are descended from people like Indians who prayed to the nature spirits, danced around trees, and played drums. If you want to understand Indians, find your own ancestral Indian first.

SUGGESTION: RECLAIM YOUR HERITAGE   Trace your heritage back as far as you can, identifying the ethnic groups and the lands from which they originate. Investigate the original nature-oriented customs, costumes, beliefs, and ceremonies of your ancestors. To cultivate your ancestral memories, research some of the traditional foods and prepare them, serving them at times of the year that were once honored by special seasonal ceremonies and festivals of that people. People who have tried this frequently find themselves starting to dream about ancient times and foreign lands that are their heritage. In some cases these dreams reveal accurate data that was previously unknown to you but that can be confirmed.

Look through old photo albums and genealogical charts for special species of animals and plants that seem to be continually associated with people in your family. Some families even have animals in their family crests, in much the same fashion that Northwest Coast Indians of North America carve totem poles to communicate their kinship ties with nature. Looking back up your family tree may reveal some nature-kinship patterns that you, too, have felt and never understood quite why. On my father's side of the family, for example, men have liked to fish as far back as I can trace.

The Sufi sequence of aligning oneself with nature, developing one's mind, and visualizing one's future proved to be an accurate predictor of my next big dream. In it I was walking along a tree-lined road in a rural countryside. Off to my left there was a grassy hill with a number of oak trees on top. This hill seemed special, and as I looked at it, it began to swell up, becoming a giant head with oak trees for hair and eyes and a mouth made from giant protruding wooden logs. The face of the earth spirit looked at me intently, and its mouth slowly opened and water began to pour out, coming toward me.

This was in 1982. Not long after the dream Rolling Thunder came to Seattle and asked me if I would like to organize a new environmental organization, the Association for Thunder People, which would bring Indians and white people together to find new spiritually based solutions to ecological problems. I knew by then that we would have to hold a dream ceremony. We did, but my dream had to do with leaving Seattle, ceasing to be a counselor, and not trying to organize the Association for Thunder People. Rolling Thunder was angry, but the dream proved to be very prophetic. A few months later Rolling Thunder's wife, Spotted Fawn, died. Shortly afterward Rolling Thunder became very ill, eventually coming down with diabetes, which cost him a foot and robbed him of his previous robust health.

Guided by dreams, in 1982 I moved to the San Francisco Bay area, which had landscapes like the one in the earth-spirit dream. The meaning of this dream was a nagging unanswered question until 1985, when the "water" began to flow. The National Audubon Society Expedition Institute asked me to organize an international symposium on the Gaia hypothesis, "Is the Earth a Living Organism?" To begin producing this event, which some administrators in the National Audubon Society declared was "two hundred years ahead of its time and will never be funded," I conducted a dream ceremony with the students and staff of the Expedition Institute. During the night of the ceremony a number of people with no prior experience in dreaming had prophetic dreams showing that the event would happen and be a success, which proved to be true a year later, when the event took place in Amherst, Massachusetts.

No sooner had I completed this program affirming the earth to be alive than dancer-choreographer Anna Halprin invited me to produce the kickoff performance of her "Circle the Earth" peace-dance program, which was based on the myths of a sacred place—my neighbor, Mount Tamalpais. The performance took place in 1986, and this peace-dance ritual is now performed in more than thirty countries around the world.

Next, psychologist Ralph Metzner invited me to produce the first conference on creating a new earth consciousness, which became the 1988 "Gaia Consciousness" conference, another first-time program. Several months later my wife and I produced our own program, the first annual Spirit of Place symposium, which brought representatives of traditional cultures together with scientists, designers, and planners to explore the modern significance of traditional earth wisdom. Throughout this process of birthing a new way of thinking about right relationship with the earth and nature, Red Feather and Mad Bear have continued periodically to appear and give useful advice, despite Mad Bear's death in the early 1980s.

Some modern theologians equate the earth spirit with the devil, witchcraft, sorcery, and evil. All of these stereotypes need to be set aside to enable nature to become a true teacher and healer. The real evil, which I came face-to-face with when I did psychiatric exams with criminals in the Seattle jail, always seemed to be linked to inner doubts, fears, and feelings of lack of self-worth. As I'll describe later, one of the best therapies for people who have become criminals and addicts seems to be immersion in nature. Nature can be cruel, but not evil. Evil seems to be more a manifestation of twisted human potential.

THE AKINA PRINCIPLE

One important lesson I've learned from following the earth spirit's guidance is that events produced according to the pow-wow tradition work on several different levels. When you follow the voices of nature, the process can take on some strange ways. I've often thought that the voice in the popular feature film *Field of Dreams* must have been the voice of the earth spirit: "Put the program together, and they will come" is what I've been hearing. Dreaming up events is not a rational process, but then nature isn't rational. Nature is a collection of systems, forces, flows, pulses, and heartbeats—all woven together into a tapestry of pure magic, just like each person. You can understand real magic only by experiencing it.

If you can accept nature as an awesome work of magic, then the laws that describe how nature works are ultimately alchemical as much as they are scientific. One of these fundamental principles of natural magic is that whenever you create a greater level of harmony in the world, the forces that have opposed that harmony will show themselves as a result, a little like an exorcism. My friend Bill Fields, retired director of Indian Affairs for the U.S. National Park Service, says that the Hopi Indians say that they don't make it rain with their ceremonies. Rather, the ceremonies drive away the disharmony that prevents the rain from falling. The Hopis call the disharmony exorcised by their ceremonies *akina.*

It's been my experience that every time I've produced an event by dreams, some kind of negative element or force that has been in hiding is exposed, exorcised by the power arising from alignment with a higher purpose. In the first living-earth symposium, as the event drew close, we received threatening phone calls from an administrator of a Massachusetts environmental group. He said he would tell all the local media we were kooks and nuts if we held the event in "his state." He felt that Massachusetts was his turf, and he did not want to lose his constituency, he said. He must have carried out his threat, because the national media carried the program widely, but the local media did not give notice of our coming or cover the event.

When I tried to run a paid classified ad in *Science* magazine for the 1989 "Spirit of Place" symposium, seeking to create a dialogue between Indians and scientists about how environmental fields might help explain Indian perception of special places, another instance of *akina* reared its head from the collective unconscious. I sent in my check for nearly five hundred dollars and didn't hear anything back from the magazine. I called *Science* to inquire, and a woman there laughed at me, saying she had my check but that such a program was "inappropriate." When I reminded her that *Science* had run ads for the "Is the Earth a Living Organism?" symposium, she replied, "That one must have slipped past us." Despite letters to the editors of *Science* from myself and Indian attorney Vine Deloria, Jr., my check was never returned, nor was the ad printed. They did not cash the check, but held it until I had to put a stop payment on it. Mechanistic science is one of the great roadblocks to living in harmony with nature. Denying that traditional people can work cooperatively with modern scientists comes close to racism and reveals how mechanistic science, by denying that spirituality and the paranormal exist, is one of the forces responsible for the destruction of the indigenous cultures of the rain forests.

Another side of this same demon appeared when the "Gaia Consciousness" program was held in San Francisco in the spring of 1988. In the same church where our meeting was being held, a group of Bay Area skeptics rented out a room for a public lecture by "The Amazing Randy," a stage magician who is one of the most outspoken debunkers of the paranormal. You can imagine the tension with half the church being filled with conservative engineers and scientists and the other half filled with Indians, Eskimos, t'ai chi teachers, artists, and humanistic psychologists. When *akina* surfaces, you render it harmless by keeping your center, not becoming afraid, and keeping connected to a higher purpose with impeccability—I've learned from experience. Modern science and ancient wisdom can serve each other, but to create an advance in human evolution, both must be willing to hold tight to the cutting edge of the blade of truth of alchemical wizardry.

The 1989 "Spirit of Place" program, "Sacred Places and Spaces," was held at Grace Cathedral in San Francisco, the largest house of worship west of the Mississippi. We were bringing together people of all races, representatives of all major religious faiths, architects, and scientists, as well as representatives of twelve different tribes of Native American Indians. When you're building a program like this, you always begin by making peace with the local spirit of place. Two weeks before the program I was delighted when my friends Lanny and Esther Pinola invited me to a special ceremony they wanted to hold in the underground ritual chamber, or *lamma,* at Point Reyes National Seashore. Lanny and Esther are of Pomo and Miwok ancestry, the indigenous tribes of the north San Francisco Bay Area, so I took this as a great honor.

Indian time works on a clock driven by forces beyond hours and minutes. When I arrived, we sat outside the holy chamber as dusk gathered, talking about the upcoming events, our intentions, and things we held to be important in life. As we talked, you could feel the *weya,* or spirit, building in the air. Periodically we could hear California valley quail calling in the bushes around us. As the *weya* intensified, the quail began flying and running out of the bushes and scurrying around the clearing. Finally Lanny said, "It's time for the ceremony now." We stood up and saw that nearly one hundred quail had formed a circle around us! "Walk quietly," Esther said, and the circle of quail moved with us as we walked across the clearing. As we went into the *lamma,* the quail were now encircling the ceremonial chamber, as if offering us protection from negative forces.

Two weeks later the program at Grace Cathedral began when Lanny and Esther brought their dance-and-song troupe into the massive Christian church. After prayers the elders began clacking out a rhythm on their elderberry clapper sticks and singing an ancient chant. The side doors opened, and in came half a dozen Indian children dancing, the boys dressed in costumes with feathered plumes that made them look just like valley quail! The girls wore flowing white scarves like the coastal fog that comes billowing in off the ocean at night, and they were carrying branches of bay leaves. They spiraled and circled the floor to the beat of melodic sounds and rhythms born in the dreamtime, and the feeling of *weya* grew very strong as invisible lines of harmony made connections of sympathy with the ceremony at Point Reyes, the indigenous plant and animal people, the Indians of that area, and the spirit of that place. Once the *akina* is driven out, real magic begins to manifest. Later several people told me they could hear a strange, deep voice of warm laughter coming from the basement under the room where the conference was taking place. "But this is the basement," I said, and then we all realized that perhaps the earth spirit was happy with the actions of this group of humans that the living earth carries on its circle journey around a golden sun.

When I shared this experience with several medicine people later, they nodded and smiled. "When all things are in harmony, the Creator speaks to us through his children," one said. I've since come to understand that once you've gone through an initial opening transcendent experience, it's as if a fire has been lit in your soul. If you care for that fire by learning to follow your intuitive guidance and performing acts of right livelihood, including service to nature and other people, special harmonies with nature are periodically struck, like lightning bolts, bridging the gap between people and nature. As a result, inner symbols and energies are activated, causing thoughts and images to bubble up to consciousness, revealing the wise creative genius in each of us that guides us to health, inspiration, and creative expression of the best kinds. The light of the flame of spirit that radiates from the eyes of tribal peoples who are living their lives in harmony with nature—above the Arctic Circle, on tiny tropical islands in the South Pacific, in isolated valleys in the Himalayas, and in the dense rain-forest jungles of Africa—is living proof of the value of achieving and maintaining nature kinship. It's little wonder that in these places we find the oldest peoples on earth.

To achieve the state of mind where true nature kinship exists and the natural world can become the most potent teaching and healing force in your life, there are two primary sources of *akina* that must be worked through: fear and guilt. The next two chapters help clear away these barriers to enable enjoyable, enriching exploration of the wilderness, where nature and human nature exist as a unitive whole.

Chapter Three

Dissolving the
Fear of Nature

Fear is the most toxic of all emotions.
Intense fear can even kill: animals,
including human beings, are sometimes
literally frightened to death.

—Carroll Izard
Human Emotions

A warm Indian-summer sun slowly moving across a sparkling-clear blue sky makes the afternoon of October 17, 1989, one of those days when the spirit of recreation prevails. At Candlestick Park in south San Francisco, the Giants and the A's are getting ready to play a game in the World Series. Fifty miles north, the Marin Waldorf school's seventh-grade class is on an overnight camp-out at Point Reyes National Seashore, and rock musician Pete Sears and I are the room parents.

At 4:00 P.M. we call the kids in from playing on the beach and begin the mile hike back to camp. A hundred yards down the road we come upon a young white-footed mouse in the middle of the road, running around in circles. We catch him easily and pet him, before putting him back in the grass so that no hawk will eat him. Another hundred yards down the road a gopher snake is crawling furiously down the road, also a risky proposition with the fall migration of hawks passing by overhead. Still farther down the trail a graceful four-point buck bursts nervously out of some bushes close by. Birds seem to be singing excitedly everywhere.

Back at camp Pete says, "Jim, get your drum and play and I'll play along on my accordion. Just play what the space feels like." I pick up my drum, close my eyes, and tune in to the vibes of the moment and begin to beat out a rhythm. There is a sense of excitement in the air, and for the next fifteen to twenty minutes everyone is dancing. At precisely 5:00 P.M. we stop, as it's time to get ready for dinner. Then, at 5:04, the whole youth hostel begins rocking like a ship on a rough sea. Getting everyone outside, we see telephone poles swaying like wheat stalks in the wind, wires vibrating like guitar strings. Fifteen seconds later the Bay Area earthquake of October 17, 1989, 7.0 on the Richter scale, has ended.

Even though we were less than a mile from the San Andreas Fault, nothing was harmed, but to the south, in San Francisco, million-dollar townhouses in the Marina district bounced up and down as if they were built on a water bed, splitting concrete foundations, buckling pavement, and toppling whole buildings. In those awful fifteen seconds a section of the Bay Bridge collapsed, and just a few miles away in Oakland twenty-four blocks of the three-tiered I-880 Cypress Freeway collapsed on rush-hour commuters. Everywhere power was out, and fires began to break out from downed electric wires and broken gas pipes. Sixty-six people died. Damage estimates exceeded ten billion dollars. Pete and I are sorry we couldn't have recorded our spontaneous performance that evening, for perhaps in that moment we were channeling the real spirit of rock and roll!

Nature is a source of great pleasure and meaning, our ultimate second lover. Nature can also be a killer, and a great generator of fear. It took two hours of group singing to get the kids to bed on that fateful October day of the Loma Prieta quake.

THE FEAR OF NATURE

Immediately following a disaster such as an earthquake, normal barriers between people dissolve. Confronted with life-and-death situations, people frequently join together in a powerful community spirit to make things happen. Some of the greatest heroes of the October 17th quake were residents along the ill-fated Cypress Freeway in Oakland, who risked their lives to climb up three tiers of badly damaged road to pull out trapped victims before police and firefighters could arrive on the scene.

Disasters can also move us to crave intimacy. Nine months later Seton Medical Center in south San Francisco reported a sudden jump of 20 to 40 percent in births—"quake babies."

As time passed, the deeper psychological effects of the quake began to well up. Shock, surprise, bravery, and compassion turned into anguish, exhaustion, despair, and grief. As people felt aftershocks ripple through the ground for weeks afterward, day and night, depression and anger developed. People can handle strong fear in large doses once in a while, but constant fear is debilitating. Right after the quake of '89, Bay Area people vented their feelings in every conversation possible, discovering that often the greatest emotional release came days and weeks after the initial shock. Gradually, for a lot of people, a burned-out numbness takes over as a result of living with the constant fear that at any time a really big quake will come. For at least six months afterward parents reported children having nightmares. Those whose homes and workplaces were damaged or destroyed were thrown into chaos as they realized their reality was shattered, and suddenly survival was no longer assured. Soon an epidemic of colds and flulike symptoms swept through the area, a by-product of the stress people felt from the quake and its devastation.

Right after the quake many shaken Bay Area residents vowed to move. Research shows that most probably won't. Natural disasters such as earthquakes appear periodically without predictable regularity. Earthquakes are more likely to occur in California due to plate tectonics, but there is no place on earth that is free from some kind of awesome, devastating natural force such as hurricanes, tidal waves, thunderstorms, volcanoes, ice storms, floods, droughts, or avalanches. Learning how to live harmoniously with nature requires us to conquer our fears of forces we cannot control, reduce their risks to us, and accept that nature cannot be controlled.

The word *fear* comes from the Old English root word *faer,* which means "sudden calamity or danger." As an emotion, fear first appears in children around six months of age. Fear of the dark or big animals is almost never found until after one and a half years and normally not until three. After age six, children become increasingly resistant to developing new fears of imaginary things. Most childhood fears of the dark, big animals, and weird imaginary-realm beings disappear by puberty, to be replaced by a whole new pantheon of fears about life, work, relationships, sex, death, and taxes. As we move through life, facing and mastering fear is one of the most central of all human emotional challenges, which is why psychologist Carroll Izard says that "fear has probably been the subject of scientific investigation more than any other emotion."[1]

When acute fear is aroused, the sympathetic nervous system goes into overdrive, pumping adrenaline to help give us extra biological arousal for safety and survival, whether you choose to fight or flee. The skeletal muscles tighten, the mouth opens, the lips draw back, and the salivary glands dry up. The heartbeat quickens, blood pressure drops due to blood being channeled to the exterior muscles, digestion shuts down, sweat beads up on your skin, and the pupils of your eyes enlarge as your field of perception narrows. When Willie Unsoeld, the great mountain climber, was asked how he could scale incredibly steep rocky outcroppings with such agility, he replied simply, "Fear is a great focalizer." The energy of fear can be channeled into the inspirational force to achieve extraordinary feats of strength and agility. It can also be turned inward into immobility and despair.

Freud showed us how fear is learned and can arise from a reaction to either external or internal sensations. Chronic fear is called anxiety, whose root is the Latin word *anxius,* which means "troubled in mind about an uncertain event." A related Greek root of *anxiety* means "press tight" or "strangle," which is an accurate description of the physiological expression of fear. People who fear sexual pleasure tighten up and may develop diseases of the sexual organs weakened by constant muscle contraction. Fear of failure is one cause of ulcers. People who fear their thoughts or feelings suffer from "anticipatory anxiety," which can be fear of fear itself. Some people who are anxious decide to use their energy by being hyperactive, perhaps flying off the handle at the least provocation. Humor is a healthy way to release nervous tension.

When a very fearful situation occurs, it can immobilize some people. In Oregon in the midseventies, an early snowstorm swept down out of the North Cascades, trapping a group of women on a survival-class outing. Faced with the reality of walking miles through a freezing blizzard, one of the women simply slumped down in tears, overwhelmed by the situation. She froze to death while others in the party who did not give in walked to safety. She died of "panic," which, ironically, is derived from the name of the nature god Pan. It's said that in the old days if you stumbled upon Pan when he was sleeping, he would shout so loudly that people could drop dead in their tracks from fright.

Imagine you are walking along a beautiful forest trail and you suddenly round a bend and come upon a giant grizzly bear. Your emotional choices fall into a continuum ranging from startle/surprise/shock to fear/terror to interest to excitement. Just how to cope best with the next few minutes is the subject of debate among wildlife experts. If a tree is nearby, you could climb it to escape the bear. Smaller, more agile black bears can climb like cats, but heavyweight grizzlies generally don't climb well at all. If you have to run very far and the bear chases you, you'll lose because a bear can outrun a racehorse for sixty yards. If by chance you're downhill of a bear, you will have a better chance in a footrace, because the animal's short front legs and longer hind legs might make it come tumbling head over heels. Some people suggest standing your ground and returning the bear's challenge by yelling, screaming, or banging on pots and pans and thus startling the animal into flight. Others suggest dropping down, playing dead, and letting the bear come up to sniff you. Still others suggest gradually retracing your steps, slowly, not making any sudden moves. If you someday find yourself face-to-face with a wild grizzly, perhaps the best advice is to do whatever you choose to do with 100 percent of what you've got. Bears seem most likely to attack you if you are indecisive. Fear can be contagious.

Some people are almost addicted to fear. They crave its adrenaline rush and seek out death-defying situations, such as skydiving, downhill skiing, white-water rafting, and hang gliding, to boost their inner juice into natural highs. When Freud spoke of the death instinct in some people, he forgot to mention the exhilaration that can come from mastering an extremely difficult challenge. Studies show that many high-risk takers are very psychologically healthy; they experience personal satisfaction and high personal esteem through mastering difficult tasks.

In all areas you can always find exceptions. An anxious downhill-ski racer came to me for counseling. He was almost good enough to make the U.S. Olympic team, but he tended to break his concentration as he approached maximum speed. "I figure if I'm going to fly downhill at nearly one hundred miles an hour, I'd better get this straightened out," he said tensely. To gain insight into his conflict, I asked him to imagine himself skiing downhill trying to break a record. He crouched and went through all the movements as he swept downhill on his imaginary run. I asked him to tell me when he felt he was beginning to break his concentration. As he reached "peak speed," his hands began to shake and he said, "Now."

I told him to hold that image, like a photo, and now imagine that he was a witness to the scene of his race. I asked him to look around in the crowd and tell me what he saw. "Shit, it's my mother watching me," he said. As we continued to explore this, he realized that he had taken up downhill racing to get revenge for her constant worrying about him. Over the next few weeks, as we explored what he really wanted to do, he came to realize that he wanted to do something for the environment, so he took his love for high-risk situations and joined Greenpeace, on the front line of civil disobedience on behalf of nature. The last I heard from him was a glowing report about having piloted a Zodiac raft in front of a Japanese whaling vessel to prevent a whale from being harpooned.

There is wise fear, which saves lives, and unwise fear, which destroys joy in life, cripples, and can kill. Not long ago, police in Marin County, California, reported a hysterical phone call from a woman who screamed she was being attacked by wild animals. With sirens blazing and guns drawn, the fleet of squad cars arrived to find raccoons raiding her garbage cans.

Fear is a primal survival impulse, but fearlessness can be learned. Hopi snake dancers pick up rattlesnakes and show no fear, empowered by the spirit. Seemingly the dancers' lack of fear is contagious to the snakes, for few bites are ever reported. Hopis say that if a dancer gets bitten, it's because he's broken concentration and allowed his fear of the snake to show.

A phobia is a fear that is out of proportion to the demands of the situation. Phobias and related anxiety disorders are the most common psychological problems in the United States. More than thirteen million people suffer from various phobias, according to the National Institute of Mental Health. Fear makes us either act out or draw inward. Recall that we do to ourselves as we do to our environment. "A neurosis is blocked

growth," Abraham Maslow pointed out, a subconscious fear
associated with something inside or outside that in reality should
not be feared. Fear is a protective emotion; it builds walls in us,
and possibly around us, to keep us from being harmed. Fear itself
isn't necessarily harmful; it can be a very valuable emotion. It
becomes a negative force when it is prolonged, cutting us off
from contact with valuable things inside and around us. One
consequence of living in a fear-plagued culture is the fortress
style of architecture and design that is rampant in most big cities.
Often what we create is a reflection of our inner reality.

Fear can either mobilize or immobilize us. What we do with
our feelings is a matter of choice and skill in knowing what to
do with emotions. If the woman with the raccoon problem were
facing raccoons with rabies, she would have had good reason to
be afraid. She could, however, have gotten rid of the healthy
animals that were frightening her by having better lids for the
garbage cans, a few mothballs sprinkled beside the cans, or by
live-trapping the racoons and releasing them at a distant location.
Instead she chose to become hysterical, as if the animals were
giant, rampaging grizzlies. Fortunately she didn't own an assault
rifle.

This poor woman suffered from zoophobia, the fear of animals. The fear of insects, entophobia, is even more common,
sometimes moving people to extreme terror, as in the Mother
Goose rhyme about Little Miss Muffet and her encounter with
the spider. Giant poisonous spiders, such as those in the movie
Arachnophobia, don't exist, but insects can cause problems, even
death. Malaria, yellow fever, bubonic plague, and Lyme disease
are just a few of the maladies insects can transfer to people. On
the other hand 80 percent of the world's food crops are pol-
linated by insects, many species of fish and birds are largely
insectivorous, and without insects we would have no honey or
silk. Even the annoying mosquito has a purpose: feeding baby
fish. Without mosquitoes, the Everglades would grow over. The
young swimming larvae are a major food source for Everglades

fish. The fish in turn are eaten by alligators, whose activity keeps channels open in the marsh. No mosquitoes, no fish, no alligators, no Everglades.

Insects are foes and friends, and we cannot afford to be swept up by irrational fears about them, because our technologies of pest control are so devastating. People in the United States spend an estimated $3.5 billion a year on insecticides and exterminators, a large part of which is precipitated by fear and not fact. Killer bees and fire ants can cause serious problems, but the Phobia Society of America reports people needing treatment who become hysterical at the sound of crickets chirping, terror-stricken at the sight of a garden spider, or frantic at the sound of a mosquito buzzing in a room. These kinds of feelings can and do get translated all too often into totally unnecessary chemical warfare, which does more harm to the rest of the ecology than the insects, because insects reproduce quickly and develop tolerance to pesticides far more quickly than bald eagles or humans do. We live in an age when it's possible to translate our inner world into very potent external realities. This power needs to be balanced by more awareness and understanding of the impact we can have on the web of life.

For many people nature is fraught with fearsome things. On a camping trip you could be eaten by bears, bitten by snakes, chased by rabid skunks, killed by avalanches, trapped in rock slides, struck by lightning, drowned by tidal waves, lost in the wilderness, frozen to death, or you could perish from thirst—all just by taking a hike. American Lake in Tacoma, Washington, has had blooms of toxic blue-green algae, which has killed cats and other animals that drink the normally pure water. Eating shellfish from ocean areas with a red-tide bloom of microorganisms can cause paralytic poisoning and even death. There are stories of a lake in Africa that periodically "explodes" from a buildup of toxic organic gases due to decaying plant materials. Nature can be deadly, but not all of nature and not all the time. Coping with fear correctly is essential to healthy psychological development. Learning is involved in nearly all fears, both in their causation and in the conquering of them.

THE DEEPER ROOTS OF FEAR

If you have deep, troubling fears about nature, or anything else, good professional psychological counseling or therapy may be the best solution. What appear to be fears of critters such as ants, bees, spiders, and bears may in fact be symptoms of psychological conflicts that lie much deeper in the unconscious. Fear of big dogs can be a child's transference of feelings about being molested by a parent. A snoopy mother can seem like a spider spinning a web you cannot escape from, which can be transferred to a fear of real spiders. Creative imagery is the language of the unconscious, as our nightly dreams remind us.

In deep probing of the psyche with thousands of people all around the world, psychiatrist Stanislav Grof finds that often unexplainable phobias are linked to traumas experienced in the earliest stages of psychological development, including before birth. These experiences, Grof feels, create conditions that can become lifelong self-limiting or self-destructive coping patterns unless they are rooted out and resolved. The manner in which phobias are linked to prenatal and perinatal experience requires much more detailed attention than can be given here. Grof's books, including *The Adventure of Self-Discovery* and *Beyond the Brain,* are definitely worth reading to get to the bottom of many kinds of fears.

The ecological imbalance we now suffer from is a reflection of our inner world, and a good deal of the problem ultimately traces back to the fear of nature. Sometimes fear makes us contract, but other times it moves us to aggression. Some modern ecological problems can be explained in terms of greed and aggression, but these, too, are ultimately conditions arising from inner insecurity: the fear of oneself. Maslow suggested that neuroses were ultimately cognitive mistakes. Many environmental problems are really outer manifestations of "ecological neuroses."

Healing a neurosis is a lot like peeling an onion. Somewhere in the wilderness of the mind there is a belief or an experience that serves as a root for a cluster of confused attitudes, beliefs, and feelings to form around. Under the right kind of life situations the cluster grows and can become a pervasive sentiment that permeates many areas of life. To heal such a complex, one starts with surface fears and then works one's way down to the very core of the problem. The geography of the fear of nature is a wilderness terrain that needs to be explored so that we can avoid falling into the quicksands, being swept away by the tidal waves, or devastated by the thunder and lightning of the mind. The following is a rogue's gallery of some of the most common nature fears.

UNRAVELING FEARS OF NATURE

THE FEAR OF MINOR IRRITATIONS

Allergies, sunburn, chills, mud, ice, rain, extreme hot and cold weather, flies, gnats, spiders, and strong winds can all decrease your enjoyment of nature and possibly lead to more serious problems. Checking the weather forecast, wearing proper clothes, and taking along proper medications should be all the precautions you need to keep simple irritations from becoming full-blown problems, such as sunstroke, hypothermia, and dehydration. Accidents can happen, and every once in a while a spider bite does come from a black widow or a brown recluse spider, but tripping in the bathroom or getting electrocuted by the kitchen blender are far more common than any consequence of being outdoors. The best preventive medicine for this kind of natural danger is common sense and keeping in good physical shape.

One of the most dramatic examples of how a whole culture can blame a harmless species for no good reason is the medieval dancing mania tarantism, which swept like a wave from Germany through Belgium, Holland, and Italy in the fifteenth century. Symptoms typically manifested as a person being taken by a "dancing fit" of wild gyrations coupled with loud shouting, screaming, and foaming at the mouth, which could continue for hours until a trance state was reached, which seemed to be a cure, at least temporarily. The word *tarantism* comes from the Italian belief that the malady was caused by a bite from a poisonous spider, for a bite from the tarantula spider will cause similar agitated symptoms.

In other places this frenzied mania was attributed to demonic possession, and the dancing sickness came to be called Saint Vitus' Dance because afflicted people often sought refuge at shrines associated with Saint Vitus or Saint John.

Psychologically speaking, Saint Vitus' Dance, or tarantism, is actually more like a mass catharsis of pent-up energies. It began right after the horrible plague of the fifteenth century, which must have roiled up considerable inner turmoil among survivors. Tarantists would sometimes report they had visions of saints and holy people when they swooned into trances following exhaustive dancing spells, which of course vented considerable pent-up emotional energy. Tarantism was actually community mental health at work.

The Italians realized the cathartic value of wild dancing and developed the tarantella folk dance, which was performed at rallies called Little Carnivals of Women because so many women took part. It was said that the spider bites could reappear once a person fell victim and that they needed to be continually "cured" for the rest of their lives by dancing, since profuse sweating is a sign that a cure is taking place.

A clue to another origin of the tarantella may be seen at Saint's Feast Day in June at Saint Paul's Chapel in Galatina, where people would come to dance, seek cures, and celebrate getting well. The celebration would begin with the invocation "My Saint Paul of the Tarantists, who pricks the girls in their vaginas; My Saint Paul of the Serpents, who pricks the boys in their testicles." At these rites many of the celebrants were celibate nuns and priests.[2]

THE FEAR OF NATURAL HAZARDS

Poison ivy, poison oak, bodies of water, cliffs, mountains, snowstorms, and quicksand—all occur in nature. Taking proper precautions of sensibility to protect yourself, a first-aid kit with medical supplies, a mirror, waterproof matches, a map, and a whistle, should be all you ever need, aside from common sense and proper clothing, to keep safe, even in wilderness areas. Not that many years ago people automatically filled in swamps if they contained mosquitoes, failing to recognize the value of wetlands as a habitat for fish and animals; and they sprayed whole communities with pesticides to control mosquitoes or gnats, even if those in the area didn't carry any diseases.

One of the most creative approaches to educating people about the false dangers of insects is the University of Illinois's annual Insect Fear Festival, which features showings of classic films including *Them!, Tarantula, Mothra,* and *The Fly,* followed by scientists who talk about fact and fiction in the insect world. Humor and fact are some of the best tools for demolishing unnecessary fears.

THE FEAR OF NATURAL DISASTERS

People who live in California should realize that an earthquake may rumble through their life at any time, and is more likely to do so than if they live in New York or Kentucky. People who live in the Midwest are more likely to have tornadoes in summer months than people who live in Anchorage, Alaska. Farmers living along the banks of the Platte River in Colorado know that flash floods happen, on an average of once every ten years to once every one hundred years, depending on how close to the river one lives.

If you live in a place where natural disasters are known to occur with some regularity, you can site your home to minimize risk, store emergency food and water, and build appropriate structures such as breakwaters and underground tornado shelters, but people don't always take such precautions. "We never thought it would happen to us" was what victims of the Bay Area quake of 1989 said over and over again. If you build a nudist colony in a swamp, it doesn't seem fair to blame the mosquitoes for biting people, yet how many rivers have been channelized with concrete because people insisted on wanting to build on the flood plain?

THE FEAR OF TOXINS — *TOXIPHOBIA*

As if the bugs aren't bad enough, a growing new fear has arisen from the attempts of modern science to keep nature at arm's length. You can't see them, taste them, see them, hear them, or feel them, but chemicals are everywhere, including in us. We know they have been disastrous to some species of animals, damaging to many more, and possibly to us, but no one seems to know quite how bad the problem is. The result is a new form of psychological disease, "toxiphobia," and a related affliction, "cancerophobia."

Jay Vroom, president of the National Agricultural Chemicals Association, says that people should be aware of the "enormous benefits and the very small risk" associated with agricultural chemicals. Despite what Vroom says, some of the chemicals commonly used in food production, such as EDB, are extremely dangerous.

Until the mid-1980s, EDB, ethylene dibromide, was applied regularly to most citrus fruits. In one tragic incident a boss at a chemical plant told one of his workers to climb into an "empty" tank that had held EDB and clean it out. The man did, and in three to four minutes he fainted from the fumes inside, falling into less than an inch of liquid at the bottom. His boss realized what had happened, climbed in to pull the semiconscious worker out, and stripped him down to spray him with water, for this deadly poison can be absorbed directly through the skin.

In ten minutes both men were unconscious, lying on the ground in their own vomit. The worker died in the emergency room minutes later, never regaining consciousness. The helicopter pilot who flew him to the hospital, all the nurses who attended him, the fire fighters, and so forth—twenty people in all—became sick soon after.

The boss also died in a few days, his body eaten up by gangrene. Then the terror began to set in as every medical person who had touched the worker or his boss became sick. The two doctors who had tried to save the men also died. So did the coroner who performed the autopsy. In all, sixty people became ill or died as a result of contact with the supposedly "clean" tank, including the former California OSHA deputy director who related this to me, Dr. Richard Wade.

Rachel Carson warned us about the dangers of toxins decades ago, but their volume is still growing. Almost 6,000 new chemical compounds are reported in the scientific literature each week. Some 55,000 new chemicals are in production. More than 3,000 have been deliberately added to foods, and over 700 have been found in drinking water. Some 12,000 pesticides with 1,200 active ingredients have been used in California. Many state fishing-and-hunting game-law booklets now carry two to four pages of cautionary warnings about places in the state where wild fish and game contain so many toxic chemicals that they aren't safe to eat, especially for children and pregnant women. Apparently there is no place left on earth where the environment is free of pesticide residues.

In a two-week period I recently clipped newspaper articles from the local paper that said: Scientists say they have found a

link between the rise in acute nonlymphocytic leukemia in children and exposure to pesticides; the Environmental Protection
Agency says pesticides may become trapped in the home for
years; and the USDA asserts that the residue rates for pesticides
in foods are the "lowest in years." Incidents such as the EDB
mass murder are rare, but no one really knows the effects of
long-term chronic exposure to modern chemicals. We are all
walking guinea pigs, and this is frightening. The good news is
that in September 1989 the prestigious National Academy of
Sciences released a report concluding, "Well-managed alternative
farms use less synthetic chemical fertilizers, pesticides and antibi-
otics, without necessarily decreasing, and, in some cases, increasing per-acre yields and the productivity of livestock systems."[3]

The symptoms of toxiphobia range from anxiety about what
vegetables to eat to full-blown paranoia. For many people the
toxiphobia is a nagging fear that they are poisoning themselves
and their children by what they eat, wear, and live in—which
unfortunately for some people is true. For others the problem
can become an almost paralyzing hysteria. We need to turn this
fear into constructive action. When mother's milk in many states
is found to contain so much PCB that it's unsafe for human
consumption, which is presently the case, it's time to stop sitting
idly by while chemical companies turn the earth into a test lab.

One of the worst aspects of toxiphobia is that it makes people
feel powerless, because only scientists are able to determine or
understand what is going on. The recent development of simple,
inexpensive test kits for radon gas in the home, and small,
relatively inexpensive magnetometers to measure electromagnetic fields, are important steps toward enabling people to clarify
how much invisible pollution is in their life.

THE FEAR OF LOSING CONTROL

I had no real idea of the fear of nature some people have until
one weekend in college when I went off camping. The camp-

ground was in northern Michigan, and I arrived in the early afternoon on Friday to ensure getting a good site before the evening crunch of work-weary Detroiters escaping from the auto industry. Pulling into the campground, I noticed that only one site was occupied. I drove around and selected my site and then went for a walk. As I approached the only other occupied site, I heard a television blaring away. On closer inspection the site was occupied by a house trailer, a boat, and a car, all arranged in a U-shape so that only the front of the site was open. It reminded me of the way western pioneers circled their covered wagons for protection against hostile Indians.

Sitting in the center of the three-sided fort was one man, in a folding chair, watching television and drinking beer. He saw me and motioned for me to come over. It turned out that he had come up the night before to get a good space for the rest of his family, who would soon be arriving. Over the next half hour he related to me how he had formed this arrangement with the boat, trailer, and car "to make it feel like home," he said, "because it gets kinda spooky out here all alone," he added nervously, focusing on the soap opera he was watching as if his life depended on it.

In a college class I taught several years ago one student made a rather dramatic life change when suddenly his heavy schedule was taken away. As a class we had been talking about alienation and reading Erich Fromm, Carl Rogers, Abraham Maslow, and Rollo May. The discussion was good, but it was entirely from the neck up, so I gave the assignment that people should not come to the next class but instead spend the three hours alone in nature contemplating their life.

In the next class after the three-hour solo many people had heartful stories to tell about how they realized they took too much for granted. People found the personal nature of the class so different and valuable that they voted to suspend the next homework assignment and instead use the normal two or three hours of reading doing something they'd always wanted to do but had never been able to find time to do before. One of the brighter students, however, was irritated. He had spent his solo time doing extra reading on alienation, he reported. As the class ended, he stormed out, saying the class was more like a party than the college education he was paying for.

When we came back together again, people had lots of great stories. The scholar, however, didn't show up for that class, nor for the next several meetings. I figured he'd dropped it for something more academic.

He reappeared the last class of the semester with a several-week-old beard and a girlfriend. He said he was quitting school and invited the entire class to a party to thank us for helping him make this decision.

At a spaghetti dinner he related how he had initially been furious about the departure from the normal schedule of reading, lecture, and discussion. He said that when he was supposed to be spending three hours thinking about his life, he plunged into more reading. But as the day came to a close, he said, he began to feel anxious. His roommate told him to go for a walk.

As the sun set over Puget Sound, his emotions began to bubble up inside. At first he felt furious that we could suspend study and just spend time thinking about life. Then as the anger waned, he began to feel frightened. This made him anxious, so he started to walk faster, which then became a run. He ran until he was out of breath, and at that moment he had the realization that he was running away from something.

He decided to hike to the top of a nearby hill and watch the moon. As he sat watching, it suddenly came to him that he'd never allowed himself to relax and do this kind of thing. In that moment he also saw himself as a frightened small boy who'd become a good student instead of growing up, pleasing his parents instead of himself.

An upwelling of anger now washed through him, and he lay down and began kicking, sobbing, and clutching tufts of grass. Somehow the phrase *earth mother* came to mind, and he made a decision in that moment that he would adopt the earth as his new mother. The rest of the night he spent on the hill talking to his new mom.

The next morning on the way back to his apartment, he met up with a girl he'd been seeing on and off whom he'd pushed away because he was too busy. She invited him into her apartment, and their relationship suddenly jumped to a new level of intensity. By the end of the day he had decided to quit school, move to another state with his girlfriend, and become an artist.

Schedules, clocks, routines, books, television, and telephones can all be valuable, and they can be as addicting as drugs or alcohol. Addiction is a way of avoiding something, which means that fear is the underlying issue.

THE FEAR OF BEING ALONE

When the U.S. military built the Dew Line Arctic radar system a few years ago, they were worried that the isolated operators of the stations would be especially susceptible to influence by seductive enemy radio broadcasts. Being "normal" today means "loading" one's mind with a lot of busy chatter, like a telephone switchboard, psychologist Charles Tart says. Without normal loading, people can become anxious, irritable, and more open to suggestion, yet all around the world spiritual aspirants have understood that revelations come more readily when one is alone in wild places, praying, fasting, and performing rituals.

There is a saying among Arab tribesmen of the Sahara that you should never approach a woman who lives alone near the desert, for she is almost certain to be an evil witch who has a spirit, or a jinni, as a lover. Others believe that people who live alone in wild places are crazy, and with some good reason. Satellites flying over wilderness areas pick up many heat blips that indicate humans living alone or in small groups—where no one is supposed to be living. Forest rangers have told me they find paranoid Vietnam vets, survivalists waiting for doomsday, smugglers, escaped criminals, and other folks similar to the cast of the *Twin Peaks* television series, who are hiding in the woods because they can't cope with society.

"Loneliness invites the powers of the Beyond, either good or evil," says the noted Jungian analyst Marie-Louise von Franz. She found this out firsthand through a wilderness solo she undertook after Carl Jung told her that isolation in wild places strengthens consciousness. This is how she described her solo:

> I thought I must try it out! . . . and so I imprisoned myself in a hut in the mountains in the snow. I felt perfectly happy because I occupied myself the whole day cooking, with what I was going to eat next, and that one pattern of behavior prevented me from getting caught by other devils. Being by nature introverted, if I went once a day to the village to get bread and milk and exchanged comments about the weather, that was quite sufficient to keep me in balance, so the effect was nil! But then I reinforced the cure and bought everything in tins so I would not have to go to the village. But I still went around skiing, so that I also stopped. Finally I forced myself . . . to sit the whole day and do nothing, to cook only very quickly cooked boring stuff—spaghetti or something like that—so that I couldn't take all my energy, and the first experience that I had was that time was beginning to drag! It dragged like hell. I sat and listened to the birds and the snow water dripping on the roof and thought I had sat an eternity but it was only ten-thirty and not yet time to cook the spaghetti, and so on, forever.

> This got worse and I stuck it out, and then the unconscious became alive because my mind got wandering on the idea that sometimes burglars got into such huts, especially escaped prisoners looking for weapons, a revolver, or civilian clothes, if they still had on their striped things. That fantasy got me completely, and not seeing that it was just the thing I was looking for, I was absolutely panic stricken. I took the axe for the chopping wood and put it beside my bed, and lay awake

trying to decide whether I would have the courage to bang such a man on the head if he came in, and I couldn't sleep. Then I had to go to the toilet which was outside in the snow in the wood, and in the night I put on my skiing trousers and went through the snow and suddenly something plopped behind me and I ran, and fell on my face, and got panting. Then I realized it was just snow which had fallen off a tree, but with my heart pumping and the axe beside my bed I still couldn't sleep.

Next morning I thought that now I'd had it and must go home, but then I had a second thought and said 'But that was what I was looking for!' Those were the devils I wanted to meet, so now I was going to make a fantasy with a burglar. I sat down and at once I saw [in my mind's eye] the burglar coming in. So I did what we call in Jungian terms an active imagination and felt absolutely fine! After that I stayed another fortnight and put the axe back and did not even lock the door. I felt absolutely safe. But whenever such a thing came up I wrote it down and dealt with it in active imagination and there was complete peace. I could have stayed weeks more without the slightest trouble, but when I met it without the means of coping with it by active imagination, I was on the right way to being nicely possessed.[4]

Von Franz's experience shows that the military's fears about the suggestibility of the lonely men working on the Dew Line were not unfounded. Yet retreat to isolation in nature is one of the most powerful transformative experiences available to man because it does enable the unconscious to be exposed.

Among the Tamang tribe of Tibet, the shaman is the *bombo*. *Bombo* psychology believes that humans have three souls. The lower soul, the *sem chang*, is centered at the solar plexus and deals with powers that are energized by anger. The first stage of spiritual development for the *bombo* calls for mastery of the lower soul, transmuting its flames upward into the second center, *yidam bhla*, the heart center, which is the soul of compassion and peace. The third soul, the *che wa,* is described as a light that arises from the head in the region between the eyes. The third soul becomes fully operational and capable of manifesting extraordinary powers when connected to the rising energies of the the first two souls.

The *bombo* pursues his quest for enlightenment by spending many hours alone in a high mountain sacred cave, called a *gufa.* When the *bombo* completes his spiritual initiation process, he is called a *gufa,* which means he has attained oneness with the high mountain cave.

Cowherds in the Alps believe that when a mountain hut has been shut up all winter, the hut become possessed by the "It," which is a combination of nature and the unconscious. If you own a summer cottage that sits vacant all winter long, you know what they mean. The place just doesn't feel right until you've cooked a meal, turned on all the lights, made a fire in the fireplace, dusted away all the corners, and made lots of loud noises.

On a vision quest, seekers typically surround themselves with a circle of stones or string, or sit on a special blanket. The purpose of creating your own space, physically and through prayers and rituals, is to defend yourself against transpersonal negativity. To get the most from the solo experience, you break down your normal ego defenses in hopes of making connections with one or more of the thousand or more realities that Buddhists say exist in parallel to temporal reality. In reaching out to become more of who you are, you seek power and this makes you potentially more vulnerable to darkness from the envy, greed, or jealousy of others, as well as visits from unwanted spirits.

This may sound superstitious, but if you think it's funny, ask a giant Japanese sumo wrestler why he insists on throwing salt around himself before entering the ring. It is for the same reason that Christ is said to have turned in circles before making important decisions: to clear away hindering transpersonal connections in order to think for himself.

THE FEAR OF TRANSCENDENCE

"All the wilderness seems to be full of tricks to drive and draw us up into God's light," John Muir proclaimed. And according to consciousness researcher Marghanita Laski, in her pioneering study of religious experiences, *Ecstasy: A Study of Some Secular and Religious Experiences,* ecstasy almost always takes place shortly after making contact with something valuable or beautiful or both. Bodies of natural water and beautiful natural scenes are among the most common environmental settings that inspire it.

The typical pattern of an ecstatic experience begins with feeling as if a force beyond yourself is guiding you to a special time and place. As you let go of your rational mind, a sense of awe and excitement occurs in which things take on a numinous quality. Then something happens—a bird sings, a gust of wind sweeps in, rain begins to fall—that triggers a shift into overdrive. Ego boundaries dissolve, and space and time as we normally know them slip away into a unitive oneness, accompanied by feelings of bliss, wonder, joy, peace, love, and truth. The experience usually lasts no more than half an hour and then fades away, but it's not forgotten.

"For those who have a religious experience all nature is capable of revealing itself as cosmic sacrality," Mircea Eliade concludes in his classic study of spiritual psychology, *The Sacred and the Profane.* Eliade's insight calls attention to how an initial transcendent experience is not an end in itself but an initiation into a new consciousness that includes a series of experiences which continuously evolve one, adding a growing perceptual richness to life and making one more appreciative of beauty and more aware of how different choices will affect one's life and destiny. The fires lit in moments of ecstasy forever after inspire a commitment to preserve and protect the natural world from which this experience originates, a pattern that can be seen over and over again in the lives of committed environmentalists.

A recent Gallup poll reported that over 30 percent of Americans say they have had at least one mystical or spiritual experience. Abraham Maslow, who researched peak experiences, felt this was probably a conservative estimate. He found that nearly all people he interviewed had had peak or ecstatic experiences, although many were reluctant to admit them. In his classic study *The Farther Reaches of Human Nature,* Maslow concluded that the frequency of having such experiences increases as people become more and more self-actualized. This finding further underscores the naturalness of the psychic bond between human beings and nature, inviting us to allow more wonder and beauty into our lives.

Letting go of their ego consciousness isn't easy for most people. It requires trust and a willingness to surrender to a power beyond oneself. Fear shields and protects the ego. Fear of nature can be expressed in a variety of ways, ranging from intellectualization and avoiding natural areas to the denial of a desire to transcend. Becoming aware of your fears of nature and allowing yourself to work through them is an essential step to permitting nature to be a teacher and a healer.

One woman reported to me that the first time she went on a wilderness solo, she became nauseated and dizzy and had to come back to camp. This experience moved her to go into therapy and come to see how she was putting a lot of energy into restraining her emotions and creative abilities. With the help of a therapist she worked through those inhibitions and a year later returned to the same solo place, where she spent several days in deep personal reflection. She emerged from this second successful solo with a much stronger sense of self-image and personal confidence, she reported.

THE FEAR OF THE POWER OF NATURE

Some of the most loved and feared characters of literature, such as Count Dracula, have the ability to change into animals when they are at their most powerful and evil. In contrast to shamanic psychologies, in which people seek to take on the qualities of animals to gain power, the modern tendency is to fear half-human/half-animal beings, believing such a state to be indicative of a rare form of mental illness called lycanthropy. The lycanthrope periodically takes on the personality of an animal, such as a wolf or a gorilla, and while in that state he or she often has extraordinary strength and violent tendencies. An exception to our aversion toward quasi-animal humans is Batman, who shows us that powers of nature can be used to serve the good. In either case, when people take on more animal qualities than human, they gain power and presence.

In the psychology of the Algonquin Indian tribe, people who become possessed by the spirit of nature are said to suffer from *windigo* or to be possessed by the *windigo* spirit. The *windigo* is a monster with a heart of ice who attacks and eats other people. *Windigo* psychosis typically appears in the dead of winter, when food is short, blood-sugar levels drop, and people are forced to stay indoors for long periods during the winter. The disease may begin with depression, nausea, lack of appetite, sleeplessness, and haunting dreams. Its ultimate manifestation is a crazed cannibal killer.

"Any effort to deny the claims of unwanted instincts can only result in the unconscious dominance of another instinctual complex," Carl Jung once wrote. The unconscious is like an inflated air mattress: Push down on one part and the other parts swell up. The raw, primal, carnal powers of nature can be terrifying and violent. Lions on the Serengeti Plain of Africa murder each other in the name of territoriality at a much faster rate per capita than humans murder in any big city or even in warfare.[5]

People sense the powers of darkness in nature, and they can

be real. Adolf Hitler was very knowledgeable about natural magic. According to Trevor Ravenscroft, in his fascinating study of Hitler's occult interests, *The Spear of Destiny,* Hitler was obsessed with the "Spear of Longinus," the spear that was used to humanely kill Jesus Christ. Supposedly whoever carries the spear is endowed with great powers and will be joined by two ravens who are guides to the Holy Grail. Hitler received instruction from a number of spiritual teachers, including the black magician Aleister Crowley, and reportedly would dress in old Teutonic costumes, go out into the woods, and perform the "berserk ceremony," which calls in the spirit of a mad bear to aid warriors in battle.

"A bit of the human soul is a leopard," Carl Jung advised, and according to the work of anthropologist Michael Harner, people can become ill and anxious if they deny their animal soul. Studying the healing methods of shamans all around the world, Harner concludes that according to shamanic psychology, illness occurs from empty spaces in consciousness. These spaces either become weak points in the mind-body system or are filled with negative energies from the person himself or from someone else. Drawing upon his extensive work with shamans, Harner has developed a guided shamanic-journey process in which people enter into trance states and search for animals to guide them. When they journey down a long tunnel and emerge into another world, they look for animal allies, which they then bring back to this world and invite to join with their bodies. The results are positive for nearly everyone who uses the Harner method, and there are numerous cases of people being healed of serious illnesses by Harner's shamanic-journey techniques described in his book *The Way of the Shaman.*

"Know the light, but keep the dark," advised the ancient Chinese sage Lao-tzu in the *Tao Te Ching.*

In the red-cedar longhouses of the Kwakiutl Indians of British Columbia, as the aromatic smoke rises from the winter fires, elders tell of the time long ago when people lived inland and in the dead of winter four young mountain-goat hunters had to defeat the dark forces of nature. Faced with starvation, the four men traveled into the heart of the wilderness to the home of *BaxbakualanuXsiwe,* the "Cannibal at the End of the World." The vicious cannibal had an insatiable craving for human flesh, feeding on humans with the dozens of open, bloody mouths covering his body. It's said that as this human-eating giant soared through the sky, the open mouths made a horrible whistling sound, a lot like the gale-force winds of the frigid British Columbia winter. And as he flew along, he had at his side two accomplices: a giant raven whose beak could crack open a man's skull and an equally large flesh-eating bird whose name translates as "crooked beak of heaven." Using their strongest magical powers, the four hunters defeated BaxbakualanuXsiwe and his two allies after a long battle and returned to the village to celebrate their triumph.

Today this myth is reenacted every winter in the *hamatsa* ceremonies, an example of primary prevention community mental health at its best. As the golden days of fall come to an end, young men who wish to become *hamatsa* go off into the woods to spend four months in isolation. During this time they fast, pray, and perform ceremonies and rituals. Then, in the dead of winter, the young men, who are crazed with a wild frenzy, are called back into the village with the blowing of high-pitched eagle-bone whistles. The initiated *hamatsas* take the neophytes and dress them in wreaths of hemlock, blacken their faces, and give them only a loincloth to wear, even though it is very cold and snow and rain are falling constantly.

The entire village assembles in the largest longhouse. Then the elder shamans, the *heliga,* wearing red headbands and scarves and shaking skull-shaped rattles that are said to have the power to control those possessed by the *hamatsa,* bring in the new initiates. Fueled by the spirit of BaxbakualanuXsiwe, the young men leap and dance about in a crazed manner. The community and the elder shamans must now unite as one mind to overpower this primal force, or the young *hamatsas* may break into the crowd and bite people, even attempt rape. After four great circles around the longhouse, the spirit of the great cannibal is tamed and the young men are now given red-cedar-bark regalia, signifying that they have been fully admitted into the order.

In celebration of their graduation the *hamatsa* dance four more times around the fire, now joined by people in costumes who depict the great cannibal and his allies. They are joined by a wildly gyrating dancer who depicts the *bookus,* or "man of the woods," who lives deep in the forest and eats rotting wood, grubs, toads, snails, and lizards. Like the bogeyman, he likes to seduce men and turn them into ghosts. In some ceremonies a "wild woman of the woods" may also appear. She is a cannibal ogress who eats children who stray away into the woods.[6]

"The power of solitude is great beyond understanding," the wizened old Eskimo shaman Igjugarjuk told the Danish explorer Knud Rasmussen during the latter's studies among the Polar Eskimos in the early 1920s. Being alone in wild places has been the inspirational touchstone for many of the world's greatest kings, artists, seers, and saints. It is a touchstone of human consciousness, but the power of nature must be treated with great respect to avoid being swept into the whirlpools of mind-nature sympathy, which can be fed by fear.

How to Dissolve the Fear of Nature

It's a bright, sunny spring day. The first wildflowers are out, and a gentle wind is blowing puffs of warm, moist air scented with honeysuckle your way. Walking down a sidewalk, you come to a wooded park with a well-defined trail covered with dry wood chips. The trail will get you to your destination just as fast as the sidewalk will. Do you want to take it, or does the thought of going into the wooded area frighten you, causing you to stay on the sidewalk? Perhaps you take the park path but find yourself ever watchful for a spiderweb that might hit you in the face. A rabbit jumps out from a pile of dead leaves, startling you. Do you recoil in fear or try to follow the bouncing white tail as far as possible?

A little farther down the path a large earthworm is crawling along, right in the middle of the path. Do you jump back in fright or stop and watch the worm go on its way?

You come upon a patch of beautiful daisies and trilliums waving in the sun. Do you bend down to smell them or hold back for fear that a bee will sting you or the flowers may activate your allergies?

Rounding a bend, you come upon a pond with several white swans swimming on it. In the distance is a snowcapped mountain, which is reflected in the pond. The scene is like a picture postcard, and the air is filled with the odors of roses blooming all around the pond. Looking at the scene, do you tighten up and move along, pushed by an imaginary schedule, or can you simply stop and drink in the beauty before your eyes, perhaps reflecting about Thoreau and his days at Walden Pond?

Fear protects us. It mobilizes us to confront danger and shields us from pain. It can also paralyze feelings and deaden the joy of life when the fear is unjustified.

A cluster of fears becomes a neurosis, which Maslow defined simply as a "cognitive mistake." To heal inhibiting fears you go slowly, one step at a time, until you can slip away the cobweb of self-imposed beliefs that keeps you from fully relaxing and enjoying contact with nature. The following exercises may be helpful to heal any fears of nature you may have.

FACE YOUR FEARS

Make a list of the ten things you'd fear most if you were hiking through a wilderness area. Just write them down without any judgments of right or wrong. Now, for each fear ask yourself why you fear this. Is it due to previous negative experiences, things you were taught as a child, your lack of familiarity with the skills necessary to master this situation (swimming, skiing, boating, and so on), or perhaps because you don't know anything about this kind of place or situation? For each fear list some steps you could take to reduce the power of this fear to prevent you from enjoying nature more—for example, learning first aid, taking swimming lessons, buying new hiking boots, buying warm clothes. This is a good exercise to use to prepare yourself for a vacation or a new place you'd like to move to or visit.

LEARN TO RELAX AT WILL

Simple procedures such as slowly taking in a breath, holding it, and then exhaling will help calm most people down. Then, to let the relaxation grow, imagine waves of relaxation washing through your body, like gentle waves moving through a tropical ocean. Imagining a cloud of golden light in front of you that you inhale with every breath can also help you to relax.

If you want to release tension, try shaking your arms and making noises and maybe adding this to movement by dancing or running. Laughter is one of the greatest ways to relax, too. Norman Cousins cured himself of a life-threatening illness by watching old slapstick movies that made him laugh. This relieved the tension in his body, which was draining his strength and keeping him from recuperative sleep.

One of the best methods of developing skills of self-relaxation and healing is autogenic training, a self-suggestion technique based on considerable medical research. *Beyond Biofeedback*, by Elmer and Alyce Green of the Menninger Foundation, is a wonderful guide to autogenic techniques and self-healing.

GIVE YOURSELF PERMISSION TO BE SENSITIVE

If you sense and feel certain things at various places, hear voices while you're walking in the woods, or see wispy shapes in the fog at twilight, don't automatically diagnose yourself as crazy and hole up indoors where it seems safe. Take note of what you sense. Use yourself as a research project. Do you sense things that seem to be coming? Do different places feel different? What impressions come to you about the future, the past, or the places you are in? Write down these impressions without any judgments. Now look at them. Are there patterns you seem to pick up better than others? Do you color your impressions in certain ways, such as being too dramatic about them, or in terms of things you are personally afraid of? Once you see patterns in your inaccuracies of prediction and sensing, you can begin to get a clearer picture of what keeps you from making the maximum use of your sensitivities, and you can then put them to use to get more enjoyment out of life.

In martial-arts training, people are taught to look at the world with "soft eyes." When people are afraid, they tend to focus on details and lose perspective of the overall process at work, which makes them become more vulnerable. The same soft eyes can also help you negotiate wild places and see more wildlife. Rather than looking at one tree or flower at a time, learn to relax and see the entire field of vision and discern the patterns. Irregularities, such as rocks in a stream, may indicate things you need to pay more attention to, but see the whole view before you focus on details. Learning to control your eyes and adjusting the way you use them can considerably reduce your fear of being in nature or in life in general.

To develop your sensing abilities, I have people imagine they have eyes in different parts of their body. Imagine that your head is in your chest, your abdomen, or your feet. What does this feel like? Move about with your eyes in each of these positions. This makes you become aware of how we unconsciously become so heady, cutting off other sensing abilities.

DEVELOP AN ACTIVE IMAGINATION

When Marie-Louise von Franz did her wilderness solo, she said she used active imagination to conquer her fears. Developing this technique is like learning to turn yourself into a movie theater. Sit in a quiet place and visualize a scene in your mind's eye that contains an element of fear, such as meeting a wild animal or paddling a boat through some rapids. Since this is in your imagination, anything can happen and you won't get hurt. To reduce your level of anxiety, the first time through just let your fear script play itself out. Let the bear eat you, the rapids pull you under, and so on. Repeat this several times until you feel the energy associated with this fear drop.

Now give yourself permission to actively engage the same scene. Again, let your fantasies go. The bear is charging you. Don't just sit there—run, climb a tree, or shoot him. The boat is swirling in the rapids. Feather your paddle, pull hard to avoid the rocks, and shoot through with a cheer. You will probably find that the first reactions will be the most aggressive—shooting the bear, jumping out of the boat, hugging a tree to keep from falling off a cliff. As you keep running the scene over and over again, you will find more and more ease in coping with the situation. The level of fear will decrease, and you will gain mastery over difficult situations, without the need to actually be there. This is the kind of imagery exercises that most professional athletes are now using to perfect their sports performance. An excellent book on the psychology of mastering various challenges in your life is *Mastery,* by George Leonard. Former University of Michigan football coach Bo Schembechler told me that every night before going to sleep he used to visualize his team winning. Bo felt this helped him keep a positive attitude, which helped him become the "winningest" coach in college football.

DESENSITIZE YOURSELF ONE STEP AT A TIME

If you are afraid of a certain situation, such as walking in the woods at night, you can reduce your fear by developing a gradual series of exercises that lead you to gently master this challenge. Start by walking through the woods in broad daylight. Now take the same path and every few feet stop and close your eyes. Learn to use your ears and nose to orient yourself, and know that you can always open your eyes if you become afraid. One of the best woods skills is learning to walk silently. An exercise to enable you to do this is to walk down a path with your eyes closed, using your feeling of the ground under your feet to help you keep your sense of direction.

Now take the same walk at twilight, maybe with a friend. The first time at night bring along a flashlight and a friend. Then do it by yourself with the light. Work yourself up until you don't need the light, maybe planning your first lightless walk on a night when the moon is full.

USE AFFIRMATIONS TO STRENGTHEN SELF-CONFIDENCE

Fears are messages we communicate to ourselves. Just as an active imagination helps you learn to control imagery, you can also gain control of the messages you give to yourself. Using an autogenic-training exercise to get yourself relaxed, develop a series of statements about how you would like to handle a certain situation and say the statements to yourself while you are in a relaxed state—for example, "I like insects," "I enjoy hiking in the mountains," "I am centered and in control of myself." Saying these affirmations to yourself will in time reprogram away negative statements of fears. Coupling these statements with imagery makes your intentions even more powerful.

If imagery, affirmations, and relaxation don't seem to work, you might want to consider getting some professional help. The

Phobia Society of America can help you find qualified people in your area. Their address is: The Phobia Society of America, 6000 Executive Boulevard, Suite 200, Rockville, Maryland 20852.

LEARN TO PROTECT YOURSELF FROM DANGERS

Keeping in good physical shape and staying healthy will reduce fear in anyone's life. A good first-aid course will also reduce your fear of being hurt in nature and feeling helpless. If you're afraid of being attacked, take a self-defense or martial-arts course. Many community education programs are available these days to help people develop nature appreciation and recreational skills. Knowledge also helps reduce fear. Fear is a great friend and teacher. If you can identify a fear, read about it, study it, face it, its control over your life will decline, and you will feel more self-confident and able to make the journey of life with more enjoyment.

*The creation of the mental realm of phantasy
finds a perfect parallel in the establishment of
"reservations" or "nature-reserves" in places
where the requirements of agriculture,
communications and industry threaten
to bring about changes in the original face
of the earth which will make
it unrecognizable.*

—SIGMUND FREUD
Introductory Lectures on Psychoanalysis

Chapter Four

ECOLOGICAL GUILT

*The psychological dangers through which
earlier generations were guided by
the symbols and spiritual exercises of
their mythological and religious inheritance,
we today must face alone, . . . as
modern "enlightened" individuals, for whom
all gods and devils have been rationalized out of existence.*

—JOSEPH CAMPBELL
The Hero with a Thousand Faces

The supermarket today is a cornucopia of choices known only to royalty just decades ago. Each week the average U.S. household makes 2.3 trips to the neighborhood grocery, each visit averaging thirty-five to forty minutes; that's about 4.3 days per year spent grocery shopping. In contrast, our hunting-and-gathering ancestors of the Paleolithic Age spent approximately twenty hours per week in pursuit of food.

The sheer amount of time people spend doing something is one indication of their focus of consciousness. Originally people worried about having enough to eat and prayed to the gods for food. When agriculture, food preservation, and transportation had advanced enough, people began worrying about eating a "balanced meal." Today, meals have become mathematical challenges of counting calories, cholesterol, fat, and fiber. More and more people are choosing organic and healthful foods, but more and more meals are eaten in the car or on the run, a granola bar or a cone of frozen yogurt replacing what once was a half-hour-long sit-down meal. Food preparation is being taken over by machines. Perhaps the most meaningful part of meals for many people today is the chance to recycle the containers after they've finished eating.

A very small percentage of people today know the experience of having blood and dirt on their hands from harvesting what they eat. In 1974 at the University of Oregon I showed a documentary film from Jerome Bruner's "Man: A Course of Study" project to a class of aspiring environmental activists. It was an accurate portrayal of traditional hunting by Eskimos driving a herd of caribou into a lake, where the hunters could overtake them in kayaks and then spear and club the animals to death. By the end of the film a number of people had rushed to the bathroom to vomit. Others were shocked at the bloody brutality, people who show no such emotions when watching a typically bloody action-adventure movie in which hundreds of people are blown to bits. Only one person in the class had ever killed an animal to eat, even though only two or three were vegetarians.

Recent studies indicate that nearly 60 percent of Americans say they feel alienated and powerless. A 1989 Louis Harris poll of 1,250 adults nationwide found that 61 percent of the people feel that "what you think doesn't count much anymore," and 39 percent of the people feel that "you are left out of things going on around you." Conventional explanations for such feelings include politics, mass media, and economics as prime causes of alienation, which is partially true. The untold story is how our loss of contact with nature is one of the most fundamental causes of alienation. And one of the most basic ways we interact with nature is by killing the food we eat.

The word *alienated* means to be removed or dissociated from something. Today in the United States, for most people the origin of food is the supermarket or the restaurant. In 1987 Americans consumed 6.896 billion pounds of fish, 35.9 million cows, 5.3 million sheep, 81.4 million pigs, 378 million chickens, and 240 million turkeys. In Japan, where there is much less space to rear land animals, 88,000 tons of mackerel are consumed each day in the city of Tokyo alone.

We think we're mobile, but what's even more mobile is the food we eat. As cold weather comes upon us, fresh vegetables come from farther and farther south, extending down into Mexico and South America. The average chicken travels 1,200 miles from where it's raised until it's on your table. Steak and hamburger journey even farther, at least 1,300 miles on the average. Maine lobsters travel across the United States, along with other transcontinental travelers, such as Alaskan king crab, New Zealand orange roughy, North Sea herring, Atlantic swordfish, and Norwegian salmon. The same is true of the lumber we build our homes with. Cutting the lawn is the closest thing to harvesting natural resources many people know from personal experience anymore. Sixty-three percent of American households say they engage in lawn care, but now we're entering the era of Astroturf. Will grass soon cease to be the only link many people have with the practice of environmental stewardship?

Imagine for a minute what would happen if the gasoline crisis of 1973–74 came back again and transcontinental transportation of food, clothing, and lumber ceased. In many ways this would be the most powerful environmental education program that could happen. Living closer to nature would be better for all of us, but the psychological issues associated with guilt could be formidable if people weren't prepared to take responsibility for the food on their table. Learning to identify plants and animals is one thing, but actually harvesting them to survive is a much different psychological experience, one that pulls you to the core of kinship with nature.

Some people oppose killing animals for any reason. Nobody seems to feel that it's wrong to kill plants, but plants are living "people" too, with feelings and even thoughts, or so I learned from the trees who used to live next to my home in Oregon. "Blades of grass scream as loud when they are being mowed as animals being killed," asserts professional tracker and wilder-ness-survival teacher Tom Brown. Cleve Backster showed us this when he hooked up his philodendron to a lie detector and proved that the emotional energy of the plant changed according to how it was treated. Vegetative intelligence is different from human intelligence, but it's still intelligence with a purpose in the overall web of life and spirit. In his moving book *The Sacred Pipe,* Joseph Eppes Brown relates what the wise Oglala Sioux seer Black Elk told him: "We regard all created beings as sacred and important, for everything has a 'wochangi'; or influence." Plant people have rights too.

If everything is alive and has consciousness—mammals, rep-tiles, birds, fish, plants, and even rocks—then performing the basic acts of living leaves us with one of the most fundamental of all psychological challenges in mastering nature kinship: We must learn to love the ultimate killer, nature, and then kill this lover to survive.

"It seems like everything I do—eating, going to the bathroom, driving a car, wearing clothes, even walking in the woods—is going to cause pollution and harm some living things," sobbed one client. She had chosen to express her guilt by becoming anorexic, starving herself to death because she could not face the truth that death and killing are essential for life to exist. Many of us have pockets of similar guilty feelings tucked away in corners of our subconscious, eating away at our enjoyment of life.

THE NATURE OF GUILT

Fear is anticipatory, having to do with a danger about to be confronted or faced, whereas guilt is a judgment of wrongdoing that punishes the actor after the act has taken place. Fear says, "Be careful, you might get hurt." The voice of guilt whispers, "You're bad," leaving behind punishing wounds to make sure you remember the lesson that you've done something you shouldn't have that has hurt something or someone or violated an ethical code of behavior.

Psychologically, guilt poisons experience. Physiologically the muscles and organs of the body involved in the guilty act don't fully relax once the experience is finished. Instead they contract in pain, storing the memory of the guilty act in the tissues as a reminder of *should*s and *should not*s, forever after becoming a sore spot that guides thought and action. More than any other organ, the stomach, our center of emotions, is the place where guilt is concentrated, as any Type-A businessman with ulcers knows. A guilty conscience can be a great driving force for workaholics.

Some guilt seems to be instinctual, especially when we hurt a loved one. Like fear, however, what makes a person feel guilty is also learned. The fear of feeling guilty is a powerful shaper of consciousness, a cornerstone of ethics and moral codes.

In general the closer we feel to the person or thing that's harmed, the greater our guilt. Breaking a human-made standard, such as getting a speeding ticket, makes you feel guilty, but paying the fine gets you off and the guilt is gone, unless it takes away the family rent money. If, while driving a car, you hit a squirrel and kill it, you may feel bad for a few minutes. Hitting and killing a deer is generally more guilt-producing. Worst of all is hitting and killing a person, at least in most cultures. In Samoa, however, traditionally murder is forgivable by performing certain rituals and giving gifts to the family of the deceased, but failing to show proper respect for the highest chiefs is not.

Psychologically speaking, only true psychopaths, such as Alfred Hitchcock's memorable Norman Bates, played by Anthony Perkins in the movie *Psycho,* feel no guilt when they kill. Thank God they're very rare.

In war, soldiers are asked to kill in the name of their country or God or both. Yet faced with pulling the trigger with another human in the sights, many soldiers toss their guns down, vomit, panic, or black out, overcome with guilt. In his book *Men*

Against Fire, Brigadier General S.L.A. Marshall reports that 15 to 25 percent of troops in combat do not fire their guns at the enemy even once.

Armies use extensive psychological conditioning to ease the burden of guilt associated with killing. According to Sam Keen, in his penetrating study of the psychology of peace and war, *Faces of the Enemy,* one of the most common motivational techniques to get people to kill others is using propaganda to make the enemy seem like an alien, a devil, a criminal, an evil person, an enemy of God, a rapist, a barbarian, or an animal or insect. Some of our early forefathers used the same psychological tactic to conquer the wilderness and the Indians.

SELF-RIGHTEOUSNESS

One day in 1700 the pious Puritan Cotton Mather was "emptying the cistern of nature and making water at the wall," when a dog came up beside him and lifted its leg, performing its own version of the act. Mather was so repulsed at this reminder of his kinship with other living creatures that on the spot he "resolved that it should be my ordinary practice, whenever I step to answer the one or the other necessity of nature to make it an opportunity of shaping in my mind some holy, noble thought." Mather also felt that forests were "dismal thickets," places where wild men and wild animals lived. (He called Indians "hounds of heaven," "agents of the devil," and worse.) To save humanity from its wildness and wilderness, Mather believed in cutting down both wild places and wild people, justifying his actions in the name of God and morality. Sexuality and wilderness have many links in the unconscious mind.

Mather's defense mechanism for avoiding feeling kinship with nature was self-righteousness, stating to oneself that one is too holy for a particular thing or thought. Righteousness has been used by many people as justification for committing horrible acts in the name of God, such as conducting the Crusades, carrying out the Spanish Inquisition, and making people into slaves. "Truth will get you to righteousness, but righteousness will never get you to truth," counsels spiritual teacher Ram Dass, a saying that should be displayed in every church. The best way to prevent feeling guilty is to know the truth and live it with heart-centered compassion. The Sufis of the Middle East say that if you have God in your heart, you can do no wrong.

In normal people, whenever guilty feelings occur, on the surface there will be shame, depression, and even despair. At a deeper level there will always be an undercurrent of anger and rage, because people don't like to feel guilty. This anger can be directed outward into aggressive behavior or turned inward into psychosomatic illness, or both. The anger is the psyche's resentment at how the memory of the guilty feeling becomes a barrier to regaining a realm of experiencing that was previously available. Deep down no one likes to feel guilty.

Self-righteousness is often a mask for old scars of unresolved guilt. Rebellion, as in the 1960s, when a counterculture advocated no restrictions on drugs, sex, or nudity, occurs when people see through the façade of self-righteousness and vent their underlying feelings of anger in a volcanic fashion. The problem with such rebellions is that they often fail to see the underlying truths in a situation and simply encourage people to act out in defiance of an authority that imposed rules rather than helped people to understand how to make healthy decisions that respect and protect life. The result is an anticulture culture, which needs for its own survival an enemy to serve as a rallying point and acts more out of defiance than from a search for wisdom. Protests against eco-disasters can help precipitate remedial action. But all too often people seem to lose sight of their reason for coming together in the first place, so that once something is accomplished, there is a great temptation among the leadership to use its power to gratify its own ends. Thus the need arises to keep finding new enemies in order to recruit followers, and the real issues become lost.

GUILT AND SELF-DESTRUCTION

When I was a psychotherapist in Seattle, a man came to me
saying, "I have cancer, cancer of the bowels and prostate, and I
know I gave it to myself." He was the son of a hellfire-and-
brimstone preacher, who always told him he was a sinner, even
if he did the smallest thing disagreeable. For good measure his
father spanked him with a Bible, to "drive the devil out of him."
He grew up with a split personality. One side had a very low
self-image, and it would do things he later regretted, including
having affairs, beating his children sometimes, and working as a
logger on a project involving the cutting of massive old-growth
Pacific rain-forest trees. These were all expressions of his underlying storm of rage for being brought up to feel guilty.

The other part of him was pious. He operated a social-service-
assistance firm that always tried to help the underdog. Many
people who saw only this side of him considered the man a real
hero. This side attempted to compensate for the burden of guilt
he otherwise felt in his life.

It became obvious after a few sessions that a war was going
on inside him between these two subpersonalities, and the physical consequence was his cancer, an explosion of malignant cellu-
lar growth fueled by this conflict. I asked him to create a fantasy
of what each of these parts of his personality might look like.
The rebellious part looked like a devil, he said. The other part
looked like a stern Pilgrim. I asked him to imagine them both
looking at each other and then interacting. He said that they
hated each other and described a violent fight going on between
them, which represented his conflict. This battle went on for
fifteen to twenty minutes, until the whole scene just exploded. As
he described this action adventure, his stomach and intestines
rumbled, and he farted loudly as years of bound-up feelings
surfaced and were channeled into his imagery.

The next scene he described was of himself as a young boy,
lying on the ground with his angry father standing before him,

barring him from a door. I asked him what he thought was behind that door. He started shaking and trembling. Then he reported that in his imagery he crawled through his father's legs and opened the door. In this new room he saw himself as a minister, which is what he'd always wanted to be but never felt right about because he felt he wasn't worthy. He left the session with tears of joy streaming down his face.

He didn't show up for his next session. I called his house. His wife said that he'd just gone to the hospital because his fever had gone up and he was in a lot of pain. I went to see him. He was weak, but he had a smile on his face. He told me to close the door. I did, and he proceeded to get out of bed. He turned around and bent over and pulled up his hospital gown, saying, "Look." On his backside there was a large, red welt. It had the shape of a hand. He stood up, turned, and said, "It looks just like what my father used to do to me. You can see his hand marks are still in me. I guess what we did brought it out."

He went on to live far past the original prognosis given him by his doctors, but he chose not to continue therapy. He simply said that he now understood what had happened, but that he'd done so many bad things during his life that he couldn't forgive himself. If he would have continued longer, he would have discovered that under the deepest layer of the guilt complex lies love, the most powerful of all human emotions and the inner root of health and healing.

Ethical standards can be translated into laws, which change guilt from a moral issue into a legal matter. When the letter of the law becomes more powerful than the spirit of the law, fear becomes more important than guilt in directing our behavior, and lawyers' battles take the place of our conscience—a very frightening situation, which breeds terrorism as a reaction to feelings of having no authority that can be trusted.

Fear is a more basic survival emotion, overshadowing guilt when dangerous situations present themselves. Living under conditions of high levels of fear, many people suspend normal codes, which are enforced by guilt, enabling them to do things they otherwise couldn't, such as in times of war. The threat of nuclear war in the world is one such force that moves people today to pay less attention to guilt about ecological exploitation. Rampant consumerism and excessive materialism are expressions of futility in the face of the terror of our age.

SELF-RELIANCE: KILLING TO LIVE

For anyone who eats meat or uses leather, killing mammals is necessary. For anyone who eats vegetables, reads the newspaper, or lives in a wooden house, killing plants, and probably insects that could eat the plants, is necessary. It's now technologically possible to live in metal and plastic homes, wear synthetic fabrics, and eat foods derived from organic chemicals. This seems to get us away from needing to kill to live, but manufacturing synthetic products entails many environmental abuses that kill. Extracting your needs from stone, you become a killer unless you feel that members of the mineral kingdom have no consciousness. Walking kills insects and earthworms. Breathing kills microbes in the air. The whole purpose of our immune system is to make us strong enough to kill off noxious microorganisms. Killing is an integral part of being alive, but for most people today the actual act of killing living things is not part of our conscious experience.

One of the most memorable people I've worked with is a Vietnam vet who had become a backwoods survivalist in the hope of healing his psychological scars of war. He had been a member of the special forces. In the heat of battle he had killed people with his bare hands and had never forgotten their screams. Coming home to a country divided about the war, he felt betrayed and confused. Born and raised on a farm, he was a crack shot and had hunted all his life. He was good enough to break a deer's neck instantly with one shot at a hundred yards. But one day a deer bolted just as he shot and he only wounded it. He had to track the animal down and kill it at close range. Standing there with the gun in his hands, the dead deer reminded him of a person he'd shot in Vietnam. Suddenly he became unglued, struck by a bolt of "guilt lightning." Contemplating suicide, he came to see me.

The Vietnam vet had grown up understanding what it means to take the life of an animal. He'd learned from his father that good hunters only kill what they need and never waste anything from wild game. He'd never found it difficult to slaughter a hog or shoot a deer, so long as it was done quickly and humanely. But now, because of his war experiences, he was hypersensitive to guilt. Guilt is an emotion easily suppressed, buried under ego control. Guilt is also cumulative. People can go along doing things they say they feel no guilt about, denying what is building up in their unconscious, until something happens where the ego boundaries loosen, such as in an experience involving shock, alcohol, drugs, or divorce, and suddenly they're overwhelmed with a volcanic eruption of old unfinished business, which can become a psychosis.

HEALING GUILT

I believe therapists tend to attract particular clients to them because they have something in common with them on an unconscious level. Earlier I told the story of my first meeting with the snow-goose people. Several months after that first dream, they returned for a second dream lesson on ecological guilt.

As the lights went up on my dream world, I was out hunting with two friends. It was a crisp November afternoon, and the dream was so vivid, I could feel the moist ground underfoot, see it as if the scene were in waking reality, and smell the damp, slightly acid, red, brown, and golden dead leaves covering the ground. Ahead we could hear a flock of geese happily cackling and honking as they fed. We got down and slowly crept up a hill.

On the other side was a massive flock of feeding snow geese. We immediately raised our guns to fire, but at that very moment a thin, veillike screen pulled up before my eyes, and I was no longer looking at white geese feeding in a field of winter wheat. Before my gun barrel was a table full of jolly men and women, sitting around large banquet tables, wearing clothes the color of the geese. I awoke from the dream with a start and barely made it to the bathroom before I threw up.

The next day I couldn't eat meat without my stomach knotting up in a ball. I wondered if the message was that I was supposed to become a vegetarian, which I had tried one time earlier but found that it made me weak and sick.

Lucid dreams don't often come from the realm of unconscious conflicts, which Freud focused on. Like bolts of lightning in a storm, dreams of the spirit world come with sudden, startling clarity, their meanings often being like koans tossed to students by an invisible Zen master.

I watched my dreams but got no further visits from the snow-goose people to help me unravel their lesson. The knot in my stomach was still there, so I decided that I needed to make contact with the birds in real life to see if that would allow me to reenter the dreamtime for more understanding.

I went to the Skagit Flats Wildlife Refuge near Bellingham, Washington, on a rainy, gray, cold December day. I performed a simple ceremony, making an offering of cornmeal, saying prayers, and singing a chant. A gust of cold north wind swept across the marsh, sending a flurry of snow that reminded me of tiny snow geese, but no geese were in sight. I retreated into a tangle of alders and cattails for shelter and took out a goose call and began blowing a hailing call. While the pattern of the notes was the same I had learned as a hunter, this time I was calling to ask for help. Finally, just at sunset, like bells on the wind, I heard faint, tinkling, high-pitched cries of snow geese somewhere above me in the snow. I began to answer them with my call, and out of the clouds appeared nearly two hundred snow geese. They made one circle of the stubble field in front of me and then spiraled down and landed. For the next few minutes I watched the scene of my dream in real life. Then, on a cue from a flock elder, they picked up and disappeared into the snow.

I walked out into the field where they had landed. Wanting to become as attuned as possible to these mysterious birds, I picked a few plantain and dandelion leaves and ate them, trying to think as I imagined a snow goose, or snow-goose person, would. At one point I found myself looking around nervously as feeding geese might do. Then I left the field, picking up a couple of white feathers that had fallen from members of the flock.

That night I lit a white candle, like the one I'd been given in my earlier dream, and laid the goose feathers all around the candle. I tossed some cornmeal at the foot of a pine tree in the yard and said prayers asking for guidance. As I was just drifting off into sleep, I slipped into a creative reverie, and suddenly a single goose flew in and landed before my eyes. The bird looked me in the eye and simply said, "You've got to figure it out for yourself." Then it flew away.

EATING WHAT YOU LOVE

Love is generally acknowledged to be the most powerful and healing of all human emotions. It causes us to appreciate and desire, try to please and protect, those whom we love. Most people would agree there are many different kinds of love, ranging from friendship to affection to the fullest passions of eros. The more we love a thing, the more we feel for it. Loving yourself and loving nature should have equal value, for at the very deepest core they are one and the same. Generally people feel the strongest about animals, then plants, then rocks and stones. But can you kill and eat what you love without feeling guilty?

Some people may self-actualize as vegetarians, but a lot of people become ill if they stop eating meat. Many people who have become vegetarians out of a sense of guilt about eating meat find themselves becoming weak, dizzy, anemic, and more susceptible to a wide variety of infections. One college-aged woman told me that as a humanitarian gesture she stopped eating meat. At first she felt good and righteous, but soon she began to develop intestinal problems and vaginal yeast infections. She tried various conventional and unconventional remedies, but nothing worked. She went home for Christmas and told her mother. Their family was of Scandinavian descent. The mother said she knew just what to do. Her remedy was to take daily long walks by the ocean, barefoot if possible, and eat fish soup. Within a month the symptoms were gone and the girl felt very healthy again. Back in school she reverted to her vegetarian diet. Within a week her illnesses came back. At that time she decided that her mother's wisdom was correct. She returned to eating meat and fish and got better.

The diagnosis of this woman's problem, according to medicine man Rolling Thunder, was that she was suffering from malnourishment because she had strayed from her ancestral diet. In general the farther from the equator your ancestry, the more meat your ancestors had in their diet. People of Scandinavian descent have lived for thousands of years on a diet high in fish. Over time your body develops a special chemical system to work with fish protein, becoming dependent on it for health. This special bioregional chemistry is passed down from one generation to the next, translated into your biochemistry, influencing the proper diet to keep you healthy. Rolling Thunder feels a person's proper diet is the diet of his or her ancestors seven generations ago.

The connection between the eating of fish and health for people in northern climates is now gaining support from the medical community. In 1989 the scientific journal *Lancet* reported a dietary study of more than two thousand men who had suffered heart attacks, conducted by Dr. M. L. Burr of the British Medical Council. In an attempt to see if diet could help reduce mortality in this high-risk group of subjects, one third were asked to eat more cereal fiber, one third were asked to eat less fat, and one third were asked to eat more fish. The low-fat and high-fiber diets had no significant effect on death rates, but "the subjects advised to eat fatty fish had a 29% lower mortality compared with those not so advised," the study reported.

MEAT: TO EAT OR NOT TO EAT

Americans today may be eating too much red meat, especially that which is high in fat. Recent studies show the average American eats more than a half pound of meat a day, and some researchers feel this high meat diet contributes to osteoporosis, obesity, kidney problems, and even possibly cancer. This is probably true, but modern stress illnesses stem more from our lifestyle, the chemicals added to meat, and the high fat content of most domestic animal meat, as opposed to the eating of meat itself. The Indian tribes of the Great Plains, who survived primarily on buffalo meat, augmented with fruits and vegetables, suffered from few of modern man's diseases when they could eat low-fat, high-protein bison meat. Eskimos traditionally have nearly all-meat diets with considerable fat and do not suffer from such "modern" diseases. Chemistry cannot explain all of life and health.

The Manichaeans, an ancient religious order founded by the Persian sage Mani, who was born in A.D. 215, forbade their followers from killing either plants or animals for food, so that they could be lifted more quickly to the light. Manichaeanism failed to capture many followers (because of starvation?), but other popular spiritual traditions of Asia forbid killing as well. *Ahimsa* is an integral concept of the Hindu, Jain, and Buddhist traditions and is a Sanskrit word that means "lacking any desire to kill." Ironically, practicing *ahimsa* doesn't necessarily mean not eating meat. The Sherpas of Nepal practice *ahimsa*, but eat meat when it's available, letting others do the killing for them.

Much the same is true of many orders of Buddhists, including the now-famous Gyuto monks, whose years of devotion enable each member of their Tibetan Tantric choir to sing three-note chords while invoking Buddhist deities. Given the opportunity to eat meat on their 1988–89 U.S. tour, the monks devoured pork chops, bacon, steaks, and poultry like snow leopards coming off a fast, so Mickey Hart of the Grateful Dead rock band (who was instrumental in bringing the monks to this country) tells me. The Sarte Monks, another Tibetan Buddhist choir, not only love meat, a friend who produced one of their concerts reports, but they also relish large quantities of ice cream!

Vegetarians like to say that two thirds of the people of the world eat little or no meat. What they forget to add is that this is partially because the countries where these people live are severely overpopulated and impoverished and there's little meat available to be eaten there. (Incidentally, some people who talk with animals tell me the animals don't like the people eating all their food.) The world today has five billion people. Many experts suggest that we should aim to reduce world population to one billion. A long-run goal for the human species must be to establish carrying capacities of human populations for each area of the world and then guide our population size to come into this number as soon as possible, and keep it there. Human contraceptive research and education is the ultimate animal-rights cause.

Shamans all around the world sometimes prescribe vegetarian diets to aid spiritual learning and to leach out toxins from the body. An all-vegetable diet will make people's consciousness more expansive and sensitive, and more prone to unitive transcendental experiences. This can be valuable when undergoing spiritual training with a master teacher, but vegetarianism can also be a sign of psychopathology. According to Jungian analyst Alfred J. Ziegler, in his insightful psychological study of illness, *Archetypal Medicine,* vegetarianism can be the first sign of progressive anorexia nervosa, which arises from a desire to escape life on the physical plane. Most of the shamanic spiritual teachers

I've met say that after students have had their initiation experiences, they should return to a diet with some meat, which will enable them to live in the material world.

The wise old shamans also say that you can only feel kinship for what you eat. Vegetarians, they say, will never understand meat eaters, such as bears, lions, eagles, and owls, because their meatless diet prevents them from attaining the same vibrational level as the carnivores and omnivores of nature. If your personal or family totem animal is a herbivore, maybe you are more naturally a vegetarian. Many of us, however, have closer ties to bears, lions, wolverines, skunks, raccoons, badgers, bears, and other meat-eating animals. Eating some meat is part of keeping kinship ties for people, if you know how to turn food gathering into a sacred act.

This doesn't mean the ten million members of the more than seven thousand animal-rights groups in the United States are wrong. We *should* ban inhumane animal-slaughtering methods such as use of the poleax and shackles and the hoisting of living animals into the air and bludgeoning them to death, which once were common slaughterhouse techniques—and are still used in some places. Some more humane methods of killing that inflict no injury or pain prior to slaughter include: (a) carbon dioxide gas—animals pass out quickly and then can be killed, usually with a knife that slits the throat; (b) electrical stunning—electrical currents shock the animals into instant comas; and (c) mechanical devices—capture bolt stunners and guns.

If we assume that all animals, including humans, have an equal right to live a healthy, happy life, then they should have the opportunity to eat the best diet for them. Here we turn to the research of Boyd Eaton, Marjorie Shostak, and Melvin Konner in one of the most important health and fitness books to come out, *The Paleolithic Prescription.* Rather than basing their diet suggestions on modern controlled studies, they look back at the evolution of human health and diet for thousands of years as anthropologists and physicians and ask what has worked best for people down through history. They find that among meat eaters in traditional cultures, diseases that modern dietary scientists link to meat eating today—cancer, heart disease, and diabetes—are virtually nonexistent.

The authors cannot find anything from the history of human evolution to support the position that meatless diets will make humans stronger, live longer, or become more humane, as some vegetarians claim. In fact they find the opposite. Meat eaters throughout history have tended to be bigger, stronger, and smarter. Some of the rest of their conclusions are as follows:

1. There is a great discrepancy between our genetic life and modern civilization. Only 1 percent of our biological makeup has appeared over the last seven million years, yet many of us live as if we had no connection to our psychic roots at all.
2. Throughout history, as meat eating has increased, people have grown taller, stronger, and healthier, at least over the last four million years.
3. Before 1900 the chief killers of humans were infections and trauma. Today the killers of modern society are heart attacks, cancer, strokes, diabetes, and hypertension—all of which are partially related to diet and were virtually unknown in earlier times. Heart disease wasn't even described as a clinical entity until 1912.
4. The flesh of wild animals is much healthier than that of domesticated ones. It has fewer calories, its fat has five times as much polyunsaturates, and it has much less fat than the flesh of domestic animals, which, in many cases, are stuffed with chemicals and confined to pens with little room to exercise.

These data all point toward the conclusion that if you really want to take better care of yourself, you should be eating more wild fish and game, for it is the ultimate health food. This either means paying premium prices at gourmet restaurants and some select markets or returning to our roots in nature by rediscovering the fisherman, farmer, or hunter in each of us and facing the fact that we must either kill to live or pay others to kill for us. To reduce our separation from nature, I'm an advocate of people learning to become conscientious killers of at least some of the food they eat.

THE HONEST KILLER, THE HYPOCRITICAL PROTECTOR

In counseling over the next several months, the Vietnam vet began to shed his burden of guilt associated with killing what he ate. We did a journey exercise to find his personal power animal, or totem, and he came up with a mink. Again, he could return to the woods and streams to hunt and to fish. These outings became a tremendous source of healing for him, restoring self-worth and giving him control over an important part of his life. Then one day he was confronted by a group of animal-rights activists who accused him of being an "inhumane killer," and who destroyed his outing by following him into the field, making loud noises to scare away game, and verbally abusing him. After this attack he sank back into a near-suicidal depression.

To my knowledge, no hunter has ever shot an animal-rights activist, which speaks highly of the character of hunters. As an old-timer once told me in a bar in northern Michigan, "Son, if you ever want to kill someone, do it in hunting season because you can always say it was an accident."

Animal-rights activists like to make inflammatory remarks, both in person and in their literature, such as those found in the pamphlet "Hunting—An Act Against Nature," distributed by the Friends of Animals organization. The pamphlet stereotypes the hunters of America as people who shoot almost anything in sight, and claims that very few of the hunters "have a real need for meat, and a big percentage can't abide the taste of wild game anyway. And any hunter who does need meat would save time and money going to the marketplace."[1]

But vegetarians are peaceful, right? Adolf Hitler and Charles Manson both practiced vegetarianism. If I had to describe how vegetarianism affects consciousness based on the behavior of many animal-rights people, I'd say that people who don't eat meat are much more angry, self-righteous, and socially disruptive than those who do. They certainly don't do their homework on who hunts or why. According to the U.S. Fish and Wildlife Service, there are about twenty-eight million licensed hunters in the United States. Studies show that hunters are well educated, more sober than baseball or football fans, and come mostly from middle- to upper-class backgrounds. Their favorite game are, in order of popularity, deer, rabbits and hares, squirrels, pheasants, quail, and doves—all of which make very good eating. If hunters truly did go out to blast any animal in sight and didn't care about eating what they shot, you'd think they would favor starlings, pigeons, crows, and rats, all of which are legal and abundant year-round in most states. Fishermen, incidentally, are twice as numerous as hunters, with nearly fifty million anglers afield one or more times a year in the U.S.

Somehow I can't see the logic of telling hunters they should buy meat at the grocery store instead of taking responsibility for killing their own food. How a slaughterhouse is more humane than a clean kill in the field escapes me. A good hunter who has to stalk and kill what he eats will have much more reverence for the meat on his table and the animal it comes from than someone whose only food gathering is selecting steaks at his local supermarket's meat counter.

Hunting is a remarkably safe sport. According to the National Shooting Sports Foundation, with a total population of nearly thirty million hunters in 1988, there were only 161 hunting fatalities, 49 of which were self-inflicted. Hunting is statistically much safer than driving a car, crossing a busy intersection in New York, living in an urban ghetto, playing tennis, jogging, or roller skating. In 1989, one hundred people across the U.S. died when deer collided with their cars. As hunting safety requirements increase and suburban deer herds skyrocket due to the absence of predators, including man, more people could conceivably be killed by deer than in hunting accidents. The Friends of Animals pamphlet goes on to declare hunting an "act against Nature on both moral and biological grounds," and it suggests that because we now live in the "age of information" people should no longer hunt.

Animals and plants should be treated humanely, with compassion and love. Doing so is part of the sacred covenant we must cultivate with the other species with which we share the earth. Market hunting is no longer legal, and poachers who slaughter animals for profit, or thrill seekers out to blast living targets for kicks, should be severely punished. Yet, on the other hand, the line of thought that argues hunting is wrong but buying meat at the supermarket is okay doesn't make sense morally or ecologically, especially when you think of the often chemically dependent lives of domesticated livestock, and the confined and environmentally destructive environment of a feedlot.

People tend to choose their social issues according to their psychological needs and conflicts. The assertion that hunting is now wrong because we live in information-rich times seems to me to be the key to understanding where the psychology of animal-rights activists goes astray.

The term *information age* comes from the best-selling book *Megatrends,* by John Naisbitt. His central thesis is that information generation, processing, and storage has become the most important fact of modern society and that we now face the danger of becoming "computer heads" who have lost touch with physical reality. Naisbitt's antidote for falling into information overload and well-informed futility is balancing high technology with "high touch" experiences to heighten human awareness of the experiences of life and its values. Without such experiences to keep us in touch with the basic rhythms and sensations of life, Naisbitt warns us, the information age will seduce us into even deeper alienation and confusion over who and what we are and what human life should be like, which will lead to self-destruction.

If you eat, you need to take lives. Killing for food is a high-touch experience that keeps us in touch with the basic needs and emotions of life and enables us to develop feelings of reverence and appreciation for life. Most hunters and fishermen take personal responsibility for the meat they eat, which makes them more honest than antihunting people who go over to a restaurant for a double cheeseburger after a hard day on the picket lines, let alone those who wear leather shoes.

Hunters today get a bum rap for many things in the past that they had little to do with, becoming targets of self-righteous guilt slingers, who most likely eat meat, fish, and vegetables, which often have not been humanely treated at all. The abuses of wildlife of the 1800s and early 1900s are well documented. Market hunting destroyed the passenger pigeon, which once darkened the skies. We nearly lost the buffalo too. While buffalo were shot for hides, meat, and tongues, it was the policy of the U.S. government to exterminate the buffalo in order to undermine the Indians, who depended on the buffalo for survival. The buffalo was nearly driven to extinction for political reasons, not blood lust among the rank and file of hunters. The exploitive hunting of the past, such as killing birds for plumes or sea otters for fur hats, is no longer legally possible.

In countries where scientific game management is practiced, lawful hunting is no longer a threat to species survival. By far the greatest threats to animals are loss of habitat, pesticides, poaching, and automobiles. In all states today these forces collectively kill several times as many animals as legal hunters, who incidentally pay more for animal-habitat preservation than anyone else through license fees.

If animal-rights people want to help wildlife, they ought to work with hunters to preserve and restore wildlife habitat, which modern civilization is ravenously gobbling up. They also ought to seek out coalitions with hunters who dislike poaching as much as the activists do and set up squads to help game wardens patrol the woods. Illegal trading in animal parts alone is an estimated

$175-million-a-year black market in the United States, much of the booty, such as bear gall bladders and deer antlers, being sold to vegetarians in Oriental countries for magical love potions and occult medicines. These are the people who are decimating animal populations, killing the largest members of the species just for one or two parts and leaving the carcass to rot. Stronger enforcement of speed laws and a requirement that everyone have ultrasonic wildlife-alerting sound devices mounted on their cars would also save countless animals' lives. These devices are now available for thirty dollars or less and alert deer to coming cars long before headlights and tire sounds. Cars killed 350,000 deer in the United States in 1989 and millions of smaller mammals and birds.

While many species of plants and animals are becoming endangered or extinct, many of the most popular game animals are more abundant than ever before, thanks to good scientific wildlife management. In a 1989 report of the U.S. Fish and Wildlife Service on animals across the country on 440 wildlife refuges that cover 92 million acres of land, wildlife biologist Dave Klinger reports, "In the 1920s there were 500,000 white-tailed deer; now there are 14 million. There were 100,000 elk; now there are 500,000. The antelope population has climbed from 25,000 to 750,000. Bald eagles (threatened most by habitat loss and pesticides) will be taken off the endangered list in the next five years."

You can find rotten eggs in every bunch, of course. Hunting is an expression of who you are, and there are some crazy hunters as well as crazy animal-rights people. The *Guinness Book of World Records* lists the second marquis of Ripon of England, who lived from 1867 to 1923, as having killed 556,000 birds in his lifetime. Perhaps in an earlier life he was the Egyptian king Amenophis III, who in the fourteenth century B.C. wrote in stone, "With my own hand, I, the Pharaoh, killed from the chariot 102 fierce-eyed lions, I killed them with my bow and spear."

Trophy hunting and fishing, where you try always to kill the biggest and strongest animals and fish, works against species vigor by taking away the most potent members of a population. Many hunters today understand this, however. Even if we could bring back all the original predators—mountain lions, wolves, grizzly bears, wolverines, and so forth—and stopped all hunting, animal populations would skyrocket, resulting in massive die-offs from diseases and lack of food. Humans have been part of the web of life as omnivores for hundreds of thousands of years. When we remove human predation from animals, often populations skyrocket and disease and famine result. Dying quickly at the hands of a skilled hunter seems a much more humane end for a white-tailed deer than starving to death in a cedar swamp in the middle of winter due to overpopulation.

Behavioral scientists are now beginning to study why people hunt. According to Steven R. Kellert of Yale University, there are three main types of hunters:[2]

1. *Meat hunters*—45.5 percent of hunters say they are out primarily to obtain meat for the winter. These people tend to be over sixty-five years old and often are retired with less income. A deer a year is a welcome addition to the diet and the budget. It saves the life of a cow and helps keep deer herds down to a level that can be supported by the available food supply.

2. *Recreational hunters*—38.5 percent of hunters are out for sport, as a hobby, to release tension. In a bar in northern Michigan your hair will stand on end when you hear guys talking about how many "sound shots" they took at noises in the woods. Others will brag about rabbits they blew apart with high-powered rifles, leaving only blood and hair left, or how many ducks, deer, or crows they've shot. For many of these people, killing is a distant, almost mechanical, act, a game played with live animals. These folks should be encouraged to vent their feelings on a shooting range or by playing volleyball. Someone who needs to pay $150 for an infrared trail monitor to give digital displays of all game that "penetrates through your zone," a product on the

market these days, is either a wildlife biologist or awfully inse-
cure.

Hunting today is not what it could be in part because it's a
pursuit that many people have forgotten about. Steaks come
from the supermarket, right? In California hunters now have to
pass a ten-hour hunter safety class to get a license. If I had my
way, I'd require people to take classes in wildlife identification
and conservation as well as firearms safety. And to boot, I'd
make everyone who wants a hunting or fishing license spend
time each year working on habitat-improvement programs. One
of the most popular classes we developed at the high school in
Ann Arbor, Michigan, in the sixties was a senior-high conservation biology class. The kids managed a one-acre pond and a
fourteen-acre woodland and shrubland as part of their class,
learning recreational skills along with basic ecological information. I'd advocate a class like that in every high school. California
now requires anyone who wants to buy a gun of any kind to wait
for two weeks after declaring his or her intent to purchase one,
which helps keep guns out of the hands of people who are likely
to misuse them. I personally prefer to hunt with a bow and
arrow whenever possible, as it requires more skill and makes me
appreciate the results even more.

3. *Nature hunters*—17 percent of the hunters enjoy being
outside and say that they have a deep "affection, respect, and
reverence" for nature. Hunters in this third category represent
the goal of restoring an honest kinship with nature. They understand the emotional experience of kinship and are willing to step
into harmony with nature and their own ancestry, to become one
with the animals they hunt, joining in one of the most basic,
primal experiences of being human.

José Ortega y Gasset described the awe of seeking your own
food thus: "When one is hunting, the air has another, more
exquisite feel as it glides over the skin or enters the lungs; the
rocks acquire a more expressive physiognomy, and the vegeta-

tion becomes loaded with meaning. All this is due to the fact that the hunter, while he advances or waits crouching, feels tied through the earth to the animal he pursues."[3]

The excitement of hunting can be an adrenaline rush for some people, but among people who are really in a sympathetic relationship with nature, the act of hunting and fishing can and does take on a mystical or spiritual quality that catapults one's consciousness back to the very roots of one's being in a way that only love, sex, and dying can. It can even be a deeply spiritual act.

MAINTAINING THE BALANCE

Ortega y Gasset eloquently described hunting magic, but he added that "every good hunter is uneasy in the depths of his conscience when faced with the death he is about to inflict on the enchanting animal."[4]

In the Sufi tradition of the Middle East they say there are seventy-two different and equally valid paths up the sacred mountain. More than one of these includes being a killer of the food we eat. The Vietnam vet I worked with finally experienced a major breakthrough when he had a series of dreams about birds of prey. Images of eagles, owls, and hawks visited him nightly, deeply inspiring him. Then one night in a dream one of the birds flew over to him and simply said, "You're one of us." Seeing the hawk as his guiding totem animal of the upper world, he surrendered to his path, which Indian psychology understands as that of a hunter, possibly even a killer under the right circumstances. The last I heard from him, he'd taken a job on a commercial fishing boat and was going to enroll in a community-college program and study to become a game warden.

In the mind of the modern person, who, as Joseph Campbell has said, has "only tentative, impromptu and not very effective guidance" about matters such as hunting and killing, guilt is the core psychological issue when it comes to delivering the lethal blow. In contrast, among traditional hunters, who have the necessary knowledge, signs, symbols, myths, and rituals to release the killer from guilt, the basic core issue is fear, for they understand that all things are ultimately connected, and the potential price for unsettling the balance of nature may come in many ways, including accidents, illness, or food shortages later on.

The continuing wisdom since the Paleolithic age asserts that each species of living thing is part of an entire family of that species, led by its elders. All members of that species in turn are linked together in a sympathetic hierarchical mind, which is additionally connected with spirit keepers in the spiritual world. Faced with the need to kill, the spiritual killer prays that the balance of nature will be with him in the hunt and that his aim will avail the animal a quick and humane death. Entering the wilderness, he offers a sacrifice to seek the support of the spirit keepers. Following the kill, the spiritual hunter shows respect for the spirit of the animal by not wasting any meat or hide and disposing of entrails in a way that respects the spirit of the deceased animal and causes no pollution. The entire ritual procedure helps ensure respect for the dead animal, its tribe, and all of nature so that the killing becomes an expression of ecological balance. If the death doesn't take place with compassion and respect for the victim and nature as a whole, the balance will be upset, and bad fortune may befall the hunter, his family, and perhaps the entire village. The spiritual hunter understands this from intuition as well as from experience and tribal laws, and approaches his work as a killer with awe, for it seems that sometimes animals actually want to help the spiritual hunter become successful.

THE WILLING VICTIM

Living among the Eskimo and Koyukon Indians of Alaska for many years, anthropologist Richard K. Nelson learned the traditional approach to hunting. Nelson reports that when he now goes hunting, deer seem to approach him as if they understand they are to be killed, causing Nelson to feel tremendous awe for and kinship with the deer he has to kill for food. In Nelson's own words, "A hunter should never let himself be deluded by pride or false sense of dominance. It is not through our own power that we take life in nature; it is through the power of nature that life is given to us."[5]

I personally have seen the willing-victim process happen with animals. On numerous occasions I've seen ducks flock to certain hunters' blinds or deer simply run out of the bushes as if they want to be shot. It happens most strongly and frequently for certain people. American Indians say such people have special "medicine" that makes this happen. So strong is this belief in Indian culture that sometimes in conversation Indians will ask "what animal" a person is to better understand his or her personality.

After witnessing a willing-victim experience, you come to understand why Eskimos and other hunting and fishing peoples believe that their tools for taking game have their own spirit. Like the *haleff*, or ceremonial knife, of the *shohet,* the Jewish ritual butcher who kills meat in the true kosher process, you come to see fish hooks, lures, and arrows as magical, possessing a spirit all their own which can aid in the successful humane taking of wild game.

SUGGESTION: Trace your family tree back at least seven generations, looking for hunting, fishing, and farming practices. Ask yourself how you would live if you were one of your ancestors seven generations ago. Referring to the methods of food gathering they used, try your hand at making a spear from a branch, a fish hook from a piece of bone, or weaving willow sticks together to make a net to catch fish. Once the tool is done, try it out and imagine what would happen if no supermarkets existed and you had to survive using such food-gathering implements.

Psychologist Danny Slomoff reports one of the most extraordinary examples of the "willing victim" in his studies of the traditional West African voodoo priest Durchback Akuete. The people of Togo sometimes sacrifice animals such as chickens and goats when certain ceremonies are performed. "This process comes from the spirits of the animals," Akuete explained. Slomoff reports that one day a chicken Akuete was going to offer in sacrifice simply squatted down on the ground when Akuete approached, rather than running off. Gently the voodoo master picked the bird up and went over to the altar to say prayers before killing it. As Akuete went into trance and began speaking with the spirits, the chicken went limp in his hands. Examination showed that the bird simply died of its own will, as if it understood that it was time to die. The voodoo priest then said that every true healer must also be a killer, for many human illnesses come from tiny microbes that must be killed in order for a person to regain health.[6] One life-form taking the life of another is one of the most fundamental of all acts of ecological balance.

The same respectful approach to hunting should also be used for plants. When picking fruits and nuts, gathering wild asparagus shoots, or collecting mushrooms after the first warm rain of spring, follow the example of the Kwakiutl woman who, when she approaches a red cedar tree to collect bark for a basket, utensils, or cloth, prays with respect to the tree as she asks its permission to take some bark,

> Look at me, my friend! I come to ask for your dress, for you have come to take pity on us, for there is nothing which cannot be used . . . I beg you this, Long-Life-Maker, for I am going to make a basket for lilyroots out of you. I pray you, friend, not feel angry with me on account to what I am going to do to you; and I beg you, friend, to tell your friends about what I ask of you. Take care, friend! Keep sickness away from me, so that I may not be killed in sickness or in war. O friend![7]

SUGGESTION: A number of experiments have now shown that talking to plants and giving them love seems to make them grow bigger and faster. If you garden, select some plants and converse with them, daily if possible, telling them why you are growing them and assuring them that you will help other plants in respect. If you don't have a garden and live in the city, you can do this with a potted plant you grow from seed (tomatoes are especially good) or by choosing some plants growing in a park.

Not everyone has "hunter or killer medicine," but we all must eat to live. Avoiding the reality that "flesh eats flesh," as Joseph Campbell puts it, prevents us from understanding and appreciating the way ecological balance works. Hubris, or false pride, was said to be the psychological dis-ease that led to the fall of the Roman Empire. When we deny and avoid facing the need to kill to live, we become victims of "ecological hubris" and fall away from ecological balance because of naïve attitudes about right relationship with nature.

No one understands the importance of "owning" your hunting medicine more than the legendary "Motor City Madman," Detroit rock-and-roll star Ted Nugent. Growing up in the streets of Detroit and Chicago, Nugent attended strict parochial schools that no doubt helped move him, like Madonna, to develop his legendary wild-man style of being outrageous as well as a skilled performer while onstage. A prodigy with the guitar (which originated from the hunting bow), Nugent began his career with the Amboy Dukes band that made him a superstar in the mid-1970s. If you read the celebrity bios of rock musicians, you'll find some people talk about Nugent's decline. His bands broke up. A first marriage came apart. Some said he was finished. Then suddenly, in 1991, he reappeared in the top ten best-selling charts with the first album by his new group, Damn Yankees.

A man with strong deer and eagle medicine, Nugent readily admits that a touchstone of motivation for his creative inspiration since the late sixties has been his "sacred time," when he's hunting with bow and arrow. Not a person to take things lightly, over the years Nugent has come to understand the importance of hunting magic, and has discovered that the more fully he speaks out about hunting as an ethical act, the more satisfaction he feels with life. So, with typical Nugent zeal, in 1990 Ted began publishing his own hunting magazine, *Ted Nugent's Bowhunter's World.* Within a year he quickly developed a thirty thousand–strong readership and found himself with a cause that seemed to lift his entire life onto a new plateau. As his mailbox swelled with letters from bowhunters, his "Damn Yankees" single was adopted by the troops of Operation Desert Storm in the Persian Gulf, and he was back to making more gold records again.

The pages of Nugent's magazine contain stories of hunting, but they also contain an ethical creed for hunters that includes the following:

> Put more into the wild than we take out, assisting in habitat conservation and helping at every opportunity.
> Restrict your bag limit even more than the law demands when animals need help.
> And strive diligently to maintain a proficiency and accuracy to optimize quick, humane kills.[8]

Another of Nugent's bylaws is to "share the wonderment of the outdoors with others, especially the young, in word and action." A man who walks his talk, through his magazine and statewide network of Michigan supporters, Ted has set up a number of stations where deer hunters can drop off hides they don't want to use. The hides are tanned and sold, with the profits going to support a summer conservation camp for kids that promotes the outdoors and archery as an alternative to drugs. As Ted says: "Life is best with our senses clear and tuned, and bow hunting is the best natural high in life."[9] (For more information on Ted Nugent's spirited outdoor magazine, see the Appendix.)

Ted Nugent, "King of the Gonzo Guitar," is a passionate,

fiery man with a heart of gold whose antics and words sometimes offend some people. Like the diversity of fall colors in a hardwood forest, hunters come in many different varieties of personality and cannot be stereotyped in any reliable fashion. In contrast, one of the great compassionate peacemakers of our times is former President Jimmy Carter, also an avid hunter and fisherman, who describes his passion for the outdoors in sometimes spiritual tones. In his autobiography, *An Outdoor Journal,* Carter says that the most vivid and pleasant memories of his early years were times when he and his father went hunting and fishing together. These outings, he says, made him feel in step with his ancestors, as well as the people of Georgia with whom he grew up. Like other presidents who have been outdoorsmen, such as George Washington, Chester Arthur, Calvin Coolidge, Herbert Hoover, Teddy Roosevelt, Grover Cleveland, Dwight Eisenhower, and George Bush, Carter often found he could do his best thinking on difficult problems in wild places. The power of nature to make him feel alive and whole is so important to him that, he admits, "during the proper seasons, the urge within me to be in the woods and fields or along a stream is such a strong and pleasant desire that I have no inclination to withstand it."[10]

As I finished this chapter, a snow goose appeared in a dream and smiled and then flew off into the sky. A few days later a friend invited me to go hunting. While the goose had smiled, I still didn't feel finished with this issue. Then another dream came. I was out hunting for deer, and a buck appeared. I raised my gun, and the deer turned into a ram, which looked at me and said "Sufi" as I shot, and I recalled the Sufi saying about having God in your heart enabling you to do no wrong. I walked over to the animal, and it turned into a man lying on the ground with a smile on his face. He said, "Before you hunt or fish, always make some kind of sacrifice, and then meditate." Then he smiled and turned into a big roast—the willing victim!

My son and I took the offer to go hunting, and on a snowy winter day we began by sitting quietly for a few minutes, attuning our minds to the swampy woodlands of northern Michigan. I offered some cornmeal, explaining why we were there. Then we let the dog be our guide. In time a rabbit jumped out of the golden marsh grass beside the frozen lake. I shot it and it went down, but kept jumping, so I shot again to make a quick kill. That night, in a dream, a rabbit ran up to me and said, "Thank you for making sure I died quickly." My wife had a similar experience with a family pet rabbit that died. She had been especially close to Pepper and suggested we bury him with a special ceremony. Despite his desire to chew the electrical cords and our furniture, we had come to love him as part of the family. We buried Pepper in the garden, placing flowers on his grave, and that night my wife had a dream in which the rabbit returned and gave her a hug with his paws.

Sitting down to a meal, after what the snow geese and deer people have taught me, I say thank you to all the creatures of nature who have allowed us to eat them. Out there someplace in the great beyond, I think I hear them saying, "Thank you," in return.

SUGGESTION: Investigate the possibility of including some wild foods in your diet. Even a few dandelion leaves in a salad strikes a harmonic chord with the place where you live, as well as tuning you to a more direct channel of natural energies and consciousness. One of the first things I learned from traditional hunters is to walk in the steps of your game for a little while in order to approach it with some of the same mind.

If you pick wild plants, remember to ask their permission first before you pick them, and know what you're picking and eating. Fishing is usually a much easier pastime to pick up than hunting and is available to nearly everyone within a few miles of home for a relatively small outlay of money. But please check your local fish and game laws and the water quality.

In order to get to know natural foods, go for a hike with a local naturalist. To get into the spirit of the occasion, try reading one of the books on natural foods by the late Euell Gibbons, who declared in his classic *Stalking the Wild Asparagus*, "There's a saving streak of the primitive in all of us."

Chapter Five

NATURE
AS TEACHER

*Trees and stones will teach
thee more than thou can learn
from the mouth of a magister.*
—SAINT BERNARD

My father was my first nature teacher. One of the first lessons
he ever taught, and one of the most important, is that you have
to have eyes and ears all over your body to really be able to
understand the world around you.

As we walked down a dirt road covered with leaves, he would
challenge me to a contest to see who could walk more quietly.
This would not only make me more aware of my feet and what
I was doing with them, but it would ask me to boost the acuity
of my hearing to become aware of very small sounds. In time I
got to where I could slip along fairly noiselessly through dry
leaves. Then he said, "Now that you make less noise than the
wind, listen for all the other animals in the forest. If you're quiet,
they'll be less cautious and make more noise."

We'd go out into the big oak-hickory woodlot that ran beside
the cattail marshes at the south end of Grosse Ile, practicing our
silent walk. When we'd get to a certain place, he'd tell me to
stand still and listen to see how many different kinds of birds and
animals I could find. Soon the *hop, hop, hop* of a feeding squirrel

becomes a very different noise from a pheasant scratching for bugs, or a house cat stalking a mouse. Birdcalls become clear, and in time you associate the voices with their makers. The noisiest animal in the woods is a domestic dog, since he doesn't need to hunt to get his food.

On the ground beneath our feet I learned that animals, too, were playing the same game of walking as quietly as possible to avoid being heard and seen, but they sometimes left signs. The sharp, clean markings of a split hoof in darker, still-moist soil meant that a deer had just been through. The distance between the pheasant's strides told us if it was running or not. Purple-black droppings filled with seeds told us the raccoons were eating wild grapes and woodbine. Clues were everywhere.

Next my father taught me how to use my eyes. If you're looking for animals, you don't look at details, at least at first. You look for patterns and breaks in the patterns. A flash of white gives away a nervous deer by the flick of its tail. Looking for ducks over a wide body of water, you scan the entire sky, looking for dark spots. Once you see something that isn't sky, then you focus and look at the wing beats. Ducks make regular, rapid wing beats. Sea gulls flap more slowly. Vultures glide with upturned wings in a V-shape. Hawks glide with wings stretched out flat on the sides. Cranes and geese look a lot alike from a distance, but if you see long feet trailing out behind, you know they're cranes. If you see long feet and slow, steady wing beats with a neck tucked in, it's a heron.

Then he taught me that animals like certain kinds of habitats. Ducks, such as scaup, redhead, and canvasbacks, dive for food and tend to be found out in deeper water, where they can find it. Mallards, black ducks, pintails, teal, and widgeon don't dive; they tip up and sift the bottom in shallow water. Squirrels prefer to live in large, nut-bearing trees, where they can also build nests in the branches or inside hollow trunks.

To increase your chances of finding what you're looking for, factor in seasonal conditions. In the Midwest, the first migratory flights of ducks in the fall are tiny teal. Then come mallards and widgeon. Then in the middle of October come the scaup, or bluebills as we called them. Later come the canvasbacks and Canadian red-legged black ducks. When snow is falling and ice forms in idle places along the shore, you can hear the whistling wing beats of goldeneye for half a mile on a quiet day. Just as the river is covering with ice, the whistling swans push through, bugling white ghosts who stick closely together in noisy flocks.

Each species has its own special desires for food and shelter and leaves its own telltale signs. With the first few warm breaths of spring the fish splashing in the marshes are spawning northern pike. Then as the water warms, giant carp invade, wallowing like hogs among the cattails as they join in group sex orgies. Finally the slender gar pike hover like logs beside weed beds, while down on the bottom ugly dogfish with mint-green bellies gorge on carp eggs. You come to understand that the gentle, unusual movement of a bullrush or the quivering of a cattail is a sign of fish underwater, and the time of the year gives you an idea of what it is.

"Experience is not what happens to you. It is what you do with what happens to you," Aldous Huxley once said. Each lake, marsh, woodlot, and field is a tapestry of possibilities for encounters with creatures that change according to the annual cycles of nature and the moods of the weather. To become a master naturalist, you learn to make yourself invisible, use your senses in special ways, understand each species and how it responds to the seasons and unique factors of place, and be at the right place at the right time.

To become a woodsman, you adopt ethics. "Never shoot a porcupine, because they are the only thing a man lost in the woods with no food or gun can catch and kill easily," my father taught me. Other cardinal rules are never to kill more than you are going to eat and never waste anything you kill, as well as following fish and game laws. People who live close to nature learn that ethical behavior helps keep the whole life process, including themselves, alive and healthy.

"It is inconceivable to me that an ethical relation to land can exist without love, respect and admiration for the land, and a high regard for its value," wildlife biologist Aldo Leopold said in what many see as the conservation bible, *A Sand County Almanac*.[1] The core of this ethic, Leopold felt, should be, "A thing is right when it tends to preserve the integrity, stability and beauty of the biotic community. It is wrong when it does otherwise."[2]

Leopold was a professionally trained conservationist, yet he reached a real turning point in his appreciation for nature when he impulsively shot a female wolf but didn't kill her. Getting close enough to administer the final shot, he looked at the old she-wolf and watched "a green fire dying in her eyes. I realized then, and have known ever since, that there was something new to me in those eyes—something known only to her and the mountain."[3]

Aldo Leopold was an environmental psychologist before the term was invented. With great insight and foresight he understood that the root cause of environmental problems is found in the human mind, asserting in 1948 that "perhaps the most serious obstacle impeding the evolution of a land ethic is the fact that our educational and economic system is headed away from, rather than toward, an intense consciousness of land."[4]

SYSTEMATIC CONNECTIONS

When I went to college and began studying natural resources, I added science to my original nature lore. Every time we studied a new plant or animal, we learned that it was not just a single creature but part of a whole taxonomic system of kingdom, phylum, class, order, family, genus, species, and variety, in English and Latin, that tied nature together into one, wondrous system. Poring over my field manuals as an undergraduate, I continually came across the name Linnaeus, which meant that the name and taxonomy of this species had been designated by perhaps the greatest naturalist of all time, Carolus Linnaeus.

Just as Copernicus, Kepler, and Newton had come along to advance chemistry and physics, so from the dark-green forests of Scandinavia arose the towering figure of Linnaeus. A physician and botanist, Linnaeus made the brilliant insight that our system for identifying creatures should not be based on how noble a creature was (in many early systems the lion was considered the most noble of animals) or how valuable it was to us for food but according to more objective criteria of its physical morphology, especially its sexual physiology. His mind was like a great computer, creating a spiderweb of associations that enabled anyone anyplace to identify a new creature by its physical characteristics. In time people from all over the world sent Linnaeus new species in hopes that he would agree they were indeed new and perhaps even name the specimen after its discoverer. Even today, his *Systema Naturae,* published in 1735, remains the definitive work in systematic biology.

A lesser-known fact about Linnaeus is that in 1732, at the age of twenty-five, he traveled 3,800 miles on foot and horseback through Lapland on special assignment for the Swedish Academy of Sciences. Linnaeus left on his journey wearing a wool coat, a round wig, and leather britches, and carrying his microscope, a net for bugs, and a rifle.

Linnaeus's diary of his journey, *A Tour of Lapland,* describes his many sightings, and periodically the notes take on a transcendental quality reminiscent of Emerson and Thoreau when he encounters great swarms of spawning fish or herds of reindeer invading his tundra camp in the night. However, Linnaeus also met with the "Indians" of the Scandinavian north, the Saami, or Lapps, who changed his life forever. His diary entries contain reveries about the healing virtues of snowmelt, the power of the sauna to cleanse the soul, and his amazement at Lapps running around nearly nude in freezing weather and catching no illness.

A portrait of Linnaeus painted on his return from Lapland shows him proudly wearing leather clothing, a strange cone-shaped hat, and carrying a Lapp shaman's drum. As his system of classification became accepted, he could not travel much because so many boxes of new specimens were being shipped to him from all over the world. However, he still taught biology, and forever after, when Professor Linnaeus would take his students on field trips, drums and horns were always sounded on departure and return, in much the same fashion that Lapp shamans might seek the blessings of the nature spirits before undertaking journeys to find reindeer.

Linnaeus never spoke too much about his spiritual transformation among the Lapps, but his reticence was no doubt influenced by the mood of the times. In the late sixth century Pope Gregory the Great instructed his missionaries to find the pagans and their worship sites, destroy the heathen idols, and erect Christian churches on the old sites. To placate the local folk, who still had the spirit of the earth in their veins and whose muscles and money were necessary to build the churches, the old numinous signs and symbols of nature—curly-horned rams, bulls, oak trees, shocks of wheat, and Pan and his consort of half-animal/half-human followers—were carved into the walls of the basements of the churches.

Later, however, the Church became less tolerant. In the eleventh century the church in England made it an offense to build a sanctuary around a tree and forbade the eating of horseflesh, both of which were seen to be acts of pagan cults. The position of the Church on nature worship was further emphasized in the witch burnings, which became popular all across Europe. Linnaeus must have carefully concealed the reason he played his drums, for in Lapland the Church forbade playing the drum, considering it an instrument of Satan.

The other great lesson I learned in college about nature came from systems theory, demonstrating that mysticism and science agree that everything is connected to everything else. The word

ecology was coined in 1869 by the German biologist Ernst Ha-
eckel, who suggested the need for a separate science of living
systems to balance reductionism. Now a household word, *ecology* is derived from the Greek root *oikos,* which means "house"
or "place to live."

While I took many ecology courses in college, the term took
on new meaning after an encounter with Margaret Mead in the
late 1960s. Mead was one of the most powerful voices for science
to become responsible for its own handiwork, especially in terms
of environmental pollution and fallout from atmospheric explo-
sions of atomic bombs. While she and Gregory Bateson worked
together on developing systems theory, it was measurements of
radioactive fallout following nuclear testing in the South Pacific
that made her acutely aware of how important systems theory
was to sound environmental management.

Mead was raised in a house where social justice and human
ethics were stressed in daily life, but her real understanding of
the potential power of human community and the beauty of
living in harmony with nature came from her fieldwork among
the traditional peoples of the South Pacific, she once told me.
"When you are far away from modern civilization's distractions,
new voices can be heard and understood," she said in a quiet,
warm voice, describing her time in Samoa as one of coming to
see how people and nature can be connected and result in so
much beauty. It's too bad that Mead had passed on when *Science*
rejected our attempt to place an ad for the "Spirit of Place"
symposium, since one of her lifelong passions was to have science help modern people understand traditional cultures and
their contribution to human evolution.

Gregory Bateson, Margaret Mead's husband for many years,
was similarly inspired by work among the tribes of the South
Pacific. In his classic *Steps to an Ecology of Mind,* Bateson presents the theory that one of the causes of mental dis-ease in
humans is the failure of modern society to take the patterns of
nature and transfer them into similar patterns of thought and

cultural organization. Bateson's theory essentially says that we've failed to become a sustainable society because we don't think ecologically, and the same faulty patterns of thinking keep us from developing an intuitive understanding of nature, creating schizophrenia as normal consciousness.

LEARNING TO SEE
INTO THE NEXT WORLD

In 1693 a retired London businessman, Izaak Walton, published a book, *The Compleat Angler.* The title sounds like that of a fishing guide, and indeed the book does contain bits and pieces of wisdom, such as "When the wind is from the south, it blows our bait into the fishes' mouth." The book, however, is largely written as a conversation among an angler, a falconer, and a hunter, which, like the modern *My Dinner with André,* covers many topics of morals, ethics, and philosophy and recognizes that encounters with nature can lift you into another dimension. One day while gazing at his bobber floating in a pool, Walton was "for that time lifted above the earth; and possest joys not promised by my birth." This experience and others moved Walton to conclude that "rivers and the inhabitants of the watery element were made for wise men to contemplate, and fools to pass by without consideration."

The power of nature to take the mind and move it into other realms was well understood by the Transcendentalist school. Ralph Waldo Emerson's sacred place was the White Mountains of New England, where "the pinions of thought should be strong." The publication of his *Nature* in 1836 ignited long-forgotten flames of nature kinship in many people, including John Muir. Emerson urged that "Man must look at nature with a supernatural eye," and when this can be done, "the greatest delight which the fields and woods minister is the suggestion of an occult relation between man and the vegetable."

Emerson's younger colleague, the brilliant Henry David Thoreau, underwent a "spiritual birth" in seclusion at his sacred place, Walden Pond. In one of the most perceptive observations about the psychology of nature kinship, Thoreau said, "The question is not what you look at, but what you see." To see implies a much deeper understanding than what the eyes alone perceive.

In the summer of 1973, while I was on my way to Alaska, I had my first lesson in seeing. Driving along a dirt road through the rugged Kluane Valley of the Yukon Territory, a vast wild land of spruce and aspen trees interlaced with willow and alder thickets beside rushing streams presided over by 19,500 feet of snowcapped Mount Logan, I came upon an Indian salmon fishing camp beside a rushing glacial river.

A run of chum salmon was under way, and the trap was churning with maroon and silver fish averaging six to eight pounds each. The Indians were taking fish from the trap as I arrived. As they neared the bottom of the trap, someone called out, "Look!" In the bottom of the trap was a giant fish nearly four feet long. At the sight of the fish, one of the older men said, "Let it go, it's an elder." They opened the gate, and the fish shot upstream like a shadow and slipped into a pool covered by a giant fallen spruce.

"You have to respect the elders in all the tribes," the older man said to me, "the plants, the animals, the mountains, the birds—they all have many tribes. If you don't respect them, you'll pay later." Overhead, several ravens chorused in support of his words, and the old man smiled.

His words brought to mind an experience I had had one day when I was nine or ten. There was a deep hole where our family's mineral well drained into a canal that emptied into Lake Erie. Approaching the hole, I saw a black, writhing swarm of bullheads four to five inches long. There must have been one hundred fish, all tightly schooling together. There was a strange feeling about the sight before me, and I did not immediately toss in my line. Almost on cue the fish on top parted, forming a circle and revealing a giant bullhead catfish nearly three feet long. For a few minutes the smaller fish held the circle, and then the whole swarm slipped off out of sight into deeper water.

Writer-attorney Vine Deloria, Jr., a member of the Standing Rock Sioux, says that people of his tribe say that events such as sighting extralarge fish—the "mother salmon" or the "mother bullhead"—are not by chance. They represent glimpses into another dimension of consciousness, where kinship ties between person and nature originate. In addition to all the human members of your family tree, according to traditional psychology each person also has familial affiliations with special stones, plants, and animals. These linkages are shared by people according to bloodlines, hence the wolf clan, the bear clan, the badger clan, the salmon clan, and so on. Among the Pacific Northwest Indians such kinship links are expressed in carved totem poles prominently displayed beside longhouses. In other tribes clan/nature kinship relationships may be be expressed in special costumes or rituals. Across the Atlantic Ocean nature relatives appear in family crests and clan badges and as decorations on utensils, musical instruments, and canoes. There is a bear on the family crest of the earl of Northumberland of England, for example. The earl supposedly had it placed there because he claimed his grandmother had been ravished by a bear, making him a direct descendant.

Some ten thousand years ago the Athepaskan Indian tribe crossed the land bridge from Siberia into North America. At the junction of the great Yukon and Koyukuk rivers in central Alaska, one band settled, which today are known as the Koyukons.

Seasoned Arctic ethnographer Richard Nelson moved into the village of Husila in 1976 to spend sixteen months living with the Koyukon, documenting natural history according to the Indians' reality. One reason he undertook his research is that despite constant hunting, fishing, and trapping pressure in this area for at least ten thousand years, there is no evidence of any species of animal or plant being forced into extinction by the Koyukons.

In his extraordinary report of his research, *Make Prayers to the Raven*, Nelson writes, "Traditional Koyukon people live in a world that watches, in a forest of eyes. A person moving through nature—however wild, remote, even desolate the place may be—is never truly alone. The surroundings are aware, sensate, personified. They feel. They can be offended. And they must, at every moment, be treated with proper respect."[5]

Only humans have a soul *(nukk'ubidze)*, but animals have a spirit, the Koyukons believe. The spirits of each plant, animal, and stone are linked together into a unity of consciousness in this world, which in turn is connected back to the spirit world, where all things begin. The origin of this cosmology dates back to the "Distant Time," long ago, when plants, animals, and people could change forms, and all were equal. When people have dreams and visions that show people and nature changing forms, they have made contact with the spirit world. Conservation practices among the Koyukon are derived from dialogues in altered states with the spirit world.

The personality and power of the spirit of each species is different, the Koyukons assert. While all have power, the wolverine, bear, lynx, otter, and wolf have the most powerful and vengeful spirits if offended. Failure to honor the spirits by not showing respect for their animal kin can result in a variety of forms of bad fortune, including accidents, food shortages, illness, and death. One shows proper respect by humane hunting and killing, making offerings of thanks to animals killed, and even bringing the animals into the home for a night before cleaning them.

In return for proper ethical behavior and respect, the animals and plants sacrificed may appear in dreams or visions or may behave unusually to become an ally and communicate special knowledge. I witnessed such a kinship tie in 1987 following a phone conversation with Rolling Thunder.

He had been ill for several years and unable to travel and give lectures. I was producing a large exposition where it was very appropriate for Rolling Thunder to appear, so I called in the hope that he had recovered. We talked for forty-five minutes, and finally he agreed to come.

After the call I walked outside for some air. There was a fig tree in the front yard of the office. Suddenly a flock of fifteen crows came to roost in the fig tree. One bird was on the top, cawing loudly, who apparently was the leader. It seemed as though he were giving instructions, since the other fourteen swooped down and landed under the tree. The leader kept up the loud cawing as he jumped from branch to branch, knocking figs down to the ground, which the crows below quickly gobbled up. While all this was going on, I was able to walk up to within ten feet of the crows. Then, all of a sudden, the flock all flew off.

Two months later, when Rolling Thunder came to town, he had fourteen people with him. He concluded his presentation with a blanket dance, where the audience formed a circle around a blanket and people were invited to place offerings of money for his helpers. All during the dance a group of drummers beat out a rhythm and chanted, and I kept thinking in my mind's eye of the forerunner of the crows in the fig tree, with Rolling Thunder "knocking out" money for his group.

One year later Rolling Thunder lost a leg as a result of a bout with diabetes. At the same time the amputation was taking place, a large limb fell off an oak tree in the yard of Mo Maxfield, one of Rolling Thunder's longtime friends. Rolling Thunder had performed many ceremonies at the foot of this oak tree whenever he came to town and would seemingly talk with the tree when he stayed at Maxfield's home. Mo reports that one day Rolling Thunder told her, "That oak tree and I are one and the same." On the day the limb fell off, no wind was blowing, Mo reports.

"Education is a process that changes the learner," George

Leonard observed in his book *Education and Ecstasy,* which remains one of the all-time most popular books written on education. In nature education we learn names, life patterns, natural history, and biology, and we sharpen our skills to sense and feel the magical world around us. The ultimate goal of learning about nature is not to master nomenclature but to bring about greater and greater sympathetic understanding of the natural world until we can enter into a knowing oneness of nature sympathy. For those who reach this state, nature becomes a teacher in return; the chemistry is much like the process of falling in love.

The Latin roots of the English word *nature* are *natura,* which means "birth," and *nasci,* which means "to be born." Educational psychologist Thomas Armstrong has pointed out, in his penetrating analysis of teaching and learning, *In Their Own Way,* that most schools have become "worksheet wastelands" driven by test-score success. Their worst failure is that they do not recognize that we learn in many different ways according to what kind of learning is needed. Drawing on brain research, psychological testing, experiments with animals, developmental work with young children, descriptive accounts of exceptional ability, and cross-cultural studies, he concludes there are seven primary styles of intelligence and learning:[6]

1. *Linguistic:* very adept with words and auditory skills, good at writing; has a good memory; makes great social scientists and writers
2. *Logical-mathematical:* strong conceptual thinkers, enjoy questioning and wondering about natural events
3. *Spatial:* thinks in visual images easily, very aware of everything around them (Eskimos are very strong in spatial awareness because of the need to deal with changing ice floes and weather conditions)
4. *Musical:* finds it easy to keep time and perceive natural rhythms, as well as discern animal sounds and calls

5. *Bodily-kinesthetic:* enjoys sports and games, hiking, climbing, and dance
6. *Interpersonal:* organizes, communicates, and leads others well; may have strong sense of empathy for plants and animals
7. *Intrapersonal:* has a strong internal world, fueled by a deep reservoir of psychic abilities, dreams, intuitions, and inner feelings

Each style of learning has its importance to the human potential, but in terms of nature being a teacher, the most important learning methods are rooted in the last two modes, interpersonal and intrapersonal perception. There are lots of good books available that deal with the first five styles of learning, but instruction in these last two is virtually nonexistent in modern society. (In traditional society, incidentally, these were the most important and well-developed modes of perception and learning.)

The following is a series of techniques aimed at helping people slip into a mode of mind where nature reciprocates the attention expressed for her creatures, and interpersonal and intrapersonal learning are more likely to occur.

STONE: A PORTAL TO MANY WORLDS

One of the great minds of natural science, Louis Agassiz, a Swiss-born Harvard professor of the mid-1800s whose naming and classification of plants, animals, and minerals was second only to Linnaeus's, understood the importance to natural science of multimodal appreciation. One geology class Agassiz offered was referred to as Stone. At the beginning of the semester Agassiz would assemble the students around a table with a pile of stones in the center. Their semester project was to take a stone and study it, reporting on it as many different ways as possible. The greater the variety of ways and the more detail with which each could be perceived, the higher the grade.

I once assigned Agassiz's "stone" as a term paper and found some unexpected results. One scholarly student spent five to six weeks diligently working on the structure, history, chemistry, geological history, and economic value of a single stone. For a grade I gave him a B. He complained, because he had compiled more pages than anyone else in the class. I told him I was willing to change his grade if he would do one more thing. "What's that?" he asked angrily.

"Let the stone talk to you," I replied.

He stormed out of the office, grumbling about my being a nut. Then, several days later, he came back looking a little bewildered. He said that he had gone home, placed the stone on his desk, swore at it, and went to bed. That night he dreamed that he flew off into space, landing on the planet Uranus. Exploring the planet's surface, he reached down and picked up something, which happened to be the stone. As soon as he had hold of the stone, its weight began to pull him back to earth. Returning to earth, he landed next to a girl he knew and realized he had an important message to tell her.

The next day, when he woke up, suddenly the stone had power. What had been an assignment was now an amulet. Instead of leaving the stone at home on his desk, as he had done before, today the stone went into his pocket. Not long after walking outside, he ran into the girl he had seen in his dream.

Needless to say, I changed his grade. He kept the stone, and later he showed me that he had part of it ground down so that he could wear it on a necklace.

NATURE AS A MIRROR: PROJECTION

Gestalt-therapy developer Fritz Perls made an enormous contribution to modern psychology when he showed that when people project themselves into the form of something else, they can obtain valuable insights and sometimes significant emotional breakthroughs. In my experience, people seem to make deeper breakthroughs when Gestalt practice is done outdoors using natural objects.

The following exercise aids the process of seeing by inviting nature to become a giant mirror for reflection.

Select a natural area where you feel safe and that feels comfortable to you. Approach the area and sprinkle a little cornmeal on the ground, at the foot of a tree if one is nearby. Say a prayer if it feels appropriate, in whatever tradition you choose. Then state your intention to the area, as if addressing a person, namely that you are there to seek guidance and kinship. Now take three deep breaths and walk in whichever direction feels comfortable to you, seeking something that seems to want to connect with you—a tree, a stone, a flower, a stream, a waterfall, and so forth. Contemplate the object. What is its mood, its personality, its qualities? Ask yourself how you are like and unlike the object.

Now imagine yourself switching roles with it, becoming it. Describe your life as that stone, waterfall, or flower as a free-form poet might recite verses spontaneously. Record these words. Now return to your self and reflect on them. How do the sentiments of this projection describe you and your reality as well as that of the object? Nature can be a great mirror of the soul.

FINDING YOUR PLANT ALLIES

In 1978, during my period of intense dreaming, I had a vivid dream one night in which an old white-haired Polynesian man appeared and told me that one day I would be working in the South Pacific on a project involving symbolism and nature. I wrote it down and forgot about it when nothing materialized in the next few months.

In 1982, when I moved to the Bay Area, my first job was working for an architectural firm. Not long after I began the job, one of the research associates received a grant from the government of American Samoa to develop its environmental-health education plan. The man had worked in Samoa for years and was very excited. That night he went out jogging, had a heart attack, and died. After some negotiating, the Samoans allowed me to take his place, making the dream begin to come true.

When I first arrived in Samoa, I spent a memorable day with Ma'a Eleasora, the water-quality control officer of the islands, who is also a *matai,* or Samoan chief. Ma'a knew I had worked with many Indian people, so he took me on a walk in the jungle to show me the plant life of Samoa. We went a short distance down the trail and came upon a tree with many ripe bananas. Ma'a stopped and said, "This is banana."

"Banana," I replied, and expected him to move on. Instead Ma'a just stood there looking at the banana tree. I became embarrassed. What was I supposed to do? Then suddenly it dawned on me that Ma'a was introducing me to a member of the bananas as a representative of that tribe of beings. I turned my attention to the cluster of pendulous yellow fruit and tried to sympathize with it. Ma'a nodded his head, and we stood there together for several minutes, not moving at all, attuning ourselves to banana consciousness. After having achieved rapport, we moved to pay our respects to papaya, palm, hibiscus, and a dozen other trees and shrubs.

Ma'a's traditional nature hike had two purposes. The first was to acquaint me with the plant life of Samoa, which is very rich and beautiful. The second was to attune me to the wisdom of the plant kingdom so that its members' wise voices would be there in the soft tropical trade winds, guiding me to develop an environmental health education that would also help preserve the Samoan culture. The plants were to be my aids and allies.

If pressed, people are usually aware of some of their allies, because they have had lifelong attractions to them—pine trees, roses, daisies, hibiscus, and so forth. If you recognize such an attraction, consider its deeper meanings. To illustrate the variety of meanings of one species, imagine that a person is attracted to a willow tree.

In Shakespeare's *Merchant of Venice,* the forsaken queen of Carthage is described as standing "with a willow in her hand, upon the wild sea-banks." The choice of the willow in this situation is based on the English folklore that willows are emblems of grief and melancholy, indicating forsaken love, for the jilted maiden wears a garland of willow.

In contrast the Greeks saw Pluto, king of the underworld, holding a willow branch in his hand, plucked from the grove of Persephone, queen of the underworld. On the island where Circe the enchantress lived, there was said to be a grove of willows decorated by corpses.

The Chinese consider the willow to be associated with immortality and, in ancient times, covered their coffins with willows. The Eskimos of some regions see willows as being the first trees; the first people emerged from the earth beside the feet of the willow. The Irish also ascribe positive magical powers to willows. The pussy willow is one of the "Seven Noble Trees of the Land" and is a charm against enchantment. The English once used the willow as a substitute for palms on Palm Sunday, seeing the water-loving tree as a symbol of freedom.

Certain trees are also said to have special powers to aid diviners. According to English legends, the five divining trees are the rowan, ash, willow, alder, and hazel. This has become translated in the willow wand, which dowsers, or water witches, use to divine underground water.

If you have such an attraction, don't jump to conclusions. Play with different interpretations until one feels right. In many cases in earlier days the special values or powers of members of the nature kingdom were carefully hidden in poetry and verse and understood only by initiates of nature religions such as the Druids, the warlocks, and the witches. In the epic poem "The Battle of the Trees" (as reported by Robert Graves in his classic study of hidden meanings in English folklore, *The White Goddess*) 237 lines of poetry are used to describe a scene of battle where species of trees are the warriors. Actually the poem is both a spell and a description of human personality types according to their plant allies.[7]

One example of the hidden sentiments is found on lines 104–107, which say,

> *The holly, dark green*
> *Made a resolute stand;*
> *He is armed with many spear-points*
> *Wounding in the hand.*

At first glance the holly would simply seem to be pictured as a tree with a warriorlike personality. However, according to some Druidic teachings, the holly can be used in spells to protect a person from evil sorcery. Since one symbol of sorcery is a hand, the meaning of these phrases then becomes that if you are being attacked by an evil sorcerer, casting a spell with a holly branch will harm the attacker's enchantment and perhaps the enchanter. This may be why it is said that the "Green Knight" carries a club of holly.

Another set of lines, 145–147, reads,

> *With nine sorts of faculty*
> *God has gifted me:*
> *I am fruit of fruits gathered*
> *From nine sorts of tree—*

The nine types of fruit trees are plum, quince, whortle, mulberry, raspberry, pear, sorb, and the black and white cherry. Graves, who had studied the ancient Irish tree alphabet, suggests that the nine fruits mentioned are really clues to the nine magic trees of Ireland: the sloe, elder, blackthorn, whitethorn, yew, oak, ash, willow, and the reed. (According to Graves the reed was seen as a tree by Irish bards because it was used to make arrow shafts.)

An even deeper meaning is that each type of tree is supposed to facilitate a certain kind of consciousness, for example, dreaming, clairvoyance, spirit communication, and so on. The power of the tree to aid such faculties stems from the belief of many nature religions that each species of tree is associated with a god or goddess, which is why herbal potions or magical spells using this species create special results. Some insights into the early herbal lore of Greece and Rome are described in the following chart based on *Green Magic,* an excellent book of European herb folklore by Lesley Gordon:[4]

CHART 6-1
SPIRITUAL ATTRIBUTES OF SOME COMMON PLANTS

Flower/Plant	Attribute	Gods/Goddesses Greek	Roman
myrtle	love	Aphrodite	Venus
olive	peace/wisdom	Athena	Minerva
vine (grape)	passion	Bacchus	Dionysus
cypress	underworld	Pluto	Dis
fir	hunt/moon	Artemis	Diana

Each person has special plant allies that help bring out various parts of the personality. The following exercise can help shed light on your affinity for plants.

Imagine yourself walking along a path. There in the path before you, you see a stone. Pick up the stone, and hold it in your hand. Look at it closely for special colors and mineral veins. Now feel its surface texture with your hand. Is it rough or smooth? Can you tell what kind of stone it is?

Now imagine you have a magical staff of power in your other hand. Hold the stone in your left hand and the staff in your right. Raise the staff up into the air and strike it down on the ground, saying, in your best magical words and thoughts, that you would like the stone to change into a seed.

Now take the seed you have created and plant it in the ground. Step back and wave your wand and watch a season pass, with snow, spring rain, and sunshine. Now the seed begins to grow. Watch it grow to maturity and note the species.

People who do this exercise to get in better touch with their vegetative soul report all sorts of plants, which often seem to be very descriptive of their personality and interests. One common plant is the sunflower. Since in many parts of the world the seeds of the sunflower are used for treating prostate trouble, I see this as an indication of a person having a calling to do healing work, often physical healing, such as massage, osteopathy, or chiropractic. Roses often appear for people with artistic calling. Vines seem to come up often for dancers, especially jazz and improvisation. Ballet dancers are more likely to find a plant such as Queen Anne's lace, or wild carrot, with lots of structure to its flowers. Architects often come up with ferns, which have definite structural qualities.

People who come up with trees tend to have leadership qualities, often with a spiritual aspect. The director of a holistic health center saw her seed become a large red maple, and she groaned at the thought of the responsibility it carried—to give comfort and nourishment to so many people. A Russian emigrant saw a larch or tamarack spring up before him. Upon questioning him, I learned he was interested in shamanism. Since the symbolic tree that Siberian shamans ascend or descend in magical-flight journeys is often portrayed as a larch, I suggested the tree also symbolized his ancestry, which he needed to study as a foundation to bring with him into the New World. Many people of Scandinavian descent report finding white birches. These tend to be sensitive people, often with good interpersonal skills. The magic lore is that the birch is a tree for purification; its branches were used for flogging lunatics, driving out the spirits of the old year in year-end ceremonies, and beating on steaming bodies as they emerged from the traditional sauna. Such people seem to often have a special calling as counselors or psychotherapists.

If you try this exercise and come up with a tree or flower that surprises you or whose meaning seems unclear, most people find it useful to trace their family tree back a few generations. Look up the folklore of nature for your ancestry, and more likely than not, you'll find some startling insights into your nature. My Scottish clan, the Gunn Clan, has the juniper as its clan plant ally. Before I learned of the clan plant, I once used a sprig of juniper as the symbol for a holistic health center I directed and had no idea why I chose this, except that it felt right.

To discover some of the deeper qualities of a plant you encounter through this exercise, some people find it useful to use a projective technique, such as having a dialogue with the plant, either in imagery or in real life. You may find this a little peculiar, but think of how many people you know who talk to their plants. You will be doing the same thing your Aunt Minnie does when she talks to her African violets, except that you will also be listening to what they say. You might also plant your special plant in your yard or in your house, as a way of ensuring that its presence is with you twenty-four hours a day.

ANIMAL ALLIES

Each of us has an inner zoo—elements of the self that express our most basic primal archetypal qualities. Plants have a strong regenerative quality, as well as a sense of permanence because of their rootedness in the soil. Animals have a strong life-force-organizing influence, defining natural personality styles. A shrewd businessman is not called a shark or a weasel for no reason. People with piercing eyes and sharp insight into the truthfulness of life are frequently referred to as eagles and owls. The recent dichotomy of attitudes toward war in military and political leaders, described as hawks and doves, is an excellent example of how we use animal imagery to describe personalities of people in common language. To get in touch with some of one's own inner animal qualities, many people find the following exercise useful.

Settle into a quiet place, either sitting or lying down. To help focus your concentration, you may find it useful to play some background music suitable for the following journey, either in a cassette player, or with a portable player with headphones. I personally like constant, steady drumming or chanting, which many tribes use to induce trance, but this is a matter of personal choice.

When you are in a comfortable place with the music playing, imagine that you are walking down a path in a special zoo, a zoo that keeps safe all those animals that are a part of you. The more vividly you can see the path, feel it under your feet, and even see and feel the wind, clouds, and vegetation of the scene, the more powerful the results will be. Most people imagine best with their eyes closed, but some people prefer to have their eyes open. Whatever works is okay.

Move down the path until you come to a large tree with steps on it, like one you may have used as a tree fort when you were a kid. This is a journey in search of personal power, so give yourself permission to wear clothes that make you feel powerful, even magical. Also give yourself permission to have a magical staff of power such as wizards have.

Look to the right of the tree. Now take your staff of power and strike it to the ground, saying, "I want to meet with the animal-spirit keeper of my right side." Look around you for what comes forward. When an animal does appear, converse with it and ask it a question or two about its nature. It represents the power and style of your masculine side.

Having struck up a relationship with this animal, now turn to the left side of the tree and again strike down your staff and ask that the guide for the left side appear. This will be your guide to the feminine aspect of yourself. Converse with it.

Now ask both animals to come forward and face each other. Observe what they do. Give them permission to work out quarrels. If they merge into one animal, this is a very strong symbol for you, suggesting a deep psychic link to this creature. Research this animal. How does it behave? What does it like? What qualities does it symbolize for you?

People who use this exercise often find themselves able to move about with greater physical ease, even grace, and be more assertive, for they feel their inner animals give them a sense of identity. They almost always report that after this exercise they feel a new affinity for animals, and many find that when going to visit a zoo or taking a hike, they have actual encounters with the animals they met in the exercise.

Painting or drawing the animals helps to integrate this exercise. If you place pictures or drawings on the walls of your home or office, the animals now become reminders of your journey. Using your imagery, you can continue your conversation with these pictures, using them as guides in much the same fashion that tribal cultures have for thousands of years. Some people also enjoy putting on music and dancing as if they are the animals. Nature kinship grows as real magic becomes more possible with new awareness and understanding.

When a rare bird is spotted, bird-watchers will go to great ends just to get a look at it, such as when a rare Ross's gull was sighted March 2, 1975, near Newburyport, Massachusetts. The bird is a pigeon-shaped gray gull, with red legs and feet and a tinge of pink on its breast. It is normally found only in northeastern Siberia, and it is rare *there*. What moves people to watch birds? Some people may just want to add another species to their life list, but psychologically speaking, the bird is a mirror of a new, previously unrealized part of yourself. Seeing a new, rare bird touches off sparks of magic inside of you, kindling ancient fires of wonder and inspiring new possibilities.

A bird from another mysterious place may also be seen as a messenger, conveying the spirit of a place the way a carrier pigeon carries messages. A shamanic interpretation of the visit of this bird might be that the people of Russia want to develop stronger ties to the United States, or that they have something important to say to us. And since the bird was a pigeonlike gull, with a tinge of pink on its breast, one might say that this visitation was a harbinger of more peaceful times to come between the United States and the Soviet Union.

A similar animal messenger appeared in Bolinas, California, in April 1990, when a male Garganey duck was spotted in a flock of blue-winged teal, also uncommon to the area. The Garganey has a brownish-purple face, dark-brown head, and a distinctive white streak above its eye. They are normally found only in Asia and Europe, so several hundred avid bird-watchers quickly gathered to see the Soviet visitor. What makes its visit so interesting is that it came just two months ahead of Mikhail Gorbachev's visit to the Bay Area, and right after a special cross-cultural exchange between Siberian and Alaskan natives.

Traditional psychology says there are no coincidences. Pay attention to unusual synchronicities you have with animals. See if they seem to correspond to any events in your life, such as certain people appearing, important events, and so on. You don't have to be a tribal person to use tribal psychology to better understand the ways in which nature is working with you to give you valuable information.

PATTERNS OF WISDOM

Buckminster Fuller said that a true principle of life could transfer across all disciplines. The followers of many esoteric sects, who spend years deep in meditation, understand this, developing mandalas or other symbols that express states of consciousness, eternal truths, and spiritual realities.

The value of Fuller's wisdom came to me personally several years ago when I was asked to edit a book about networking. I wanted to do the project, but found that almost immediately I developed a writing block. After a couple of weeks of frustration I decided to consult with the nature kingdom for guidance. I went to a favorite place in the nearby Golden Gate Recreation Area, where I made an offering of cornmeal, sang a prayer song, and then began to wander. Within five minutes I felt pulled to a particular spot that didn't really seem that different from its surroundings. I looked and looked and couldn't figure out what was going on. Then suddenly I saw that there was a spider at work weaving a web. I watched the spider for a few moments, and then it dawned on me that this was the original network builder at work. For the next half hour I watched that spider finish its web, noting how it carefully laid out the structure and then wove it together with great patience and attention to pattern. I went home, drew a picture of the spider, and put it over my typewriter. Almost immediately the ideas began to flow and the book took form, inspired by the original networkers.

The power of symbols like the ones that arise from these exercises is sometimes challenged by politically active environmentalists as being a waste of time. Below the level of the conscious mind there is nothing but energies and symbols. Know how to work with symbols and you'll know how to sway the minds of millions. No one understood this more than one of the more powerful environmentalists of our time, Walt Disney, who was born into a modest Chicago household on December 5, 1901. In 1906 Elias Disney, Walt's father, moved the family to a forty-eight-acre farm outside Marceline, Missouri. Stimulated by nature, Disney began to draw, beginning a career that spawned lovable Mickey Mouse, Donald Duck, masterful animations of fairy tales, television shows, nature movies, and some of the most innovative amusement parks ever built—personally touching the lives of children of all ages all around the world. Disney, incidentally, is a perfect example of the fact that schools often have difficulty with creative genius; he never finished high school and only took a few formal art lessons.

The EPCOT Center in Florida, still under construction at Disney's death in 1964, was not just Disneyland East to Walt. EPCOT stands for "Experimental Prototype Community of Tomorrow." Alarmed by the world's environmental problems, Disney saw EPCOT as a place for experimenting with "new ideas of new technologies emerging from the creative centers of American industry," which could provide solutions to ecological dilemmas.[9]

NATURE SPIRITUALITY AND SPIRITS

"The nature spirits are never dead, they are alive under our feet, over our heads, all around us, ready to speak when we are silent and centered," asserts Gary Snyder in his poetic book *Good, Wild, Sacred.* Poets enjoy license to say bold things that scientists can only dream about.

When people report seeing things or hearing voices, modern psychology says these phenomena are *always* projections of inner reality, creative interpretations of experience using symbolic language or hallucinations, which may mean psychosis. Tribal psychology does not deny the existence of inner reality, but it also believes in the existence of a collective intelligence that extends beyond the physical boundaries of material reality—this means spirits.

The word *spirit* comes from the Latin *spirare,* which means "to breathe." Spirit is something you understand at a pep rally or town hall meeting when a spontaneous wave of energy swells up from the crowd into a roaring, hand-clapping cheer. "Spirits" are supernatural beings without material bodies. In the folklore of every country around the world there are spirits of various types who dwell in wild places, beside springs, under bridges, and in groves of old trees. They are some of the most common and valuable nature teachers, according to bush psychology.

According to West African voodoo priest Durchback Akuete, when he enters a trance in a ceremony and invokes spirits, he can send them to help people by pointing in the direction that he wants the spirit to go and blowing across one of his fingers. The son of a deeply religious Christian family, Akuete often demonstrated paranormal powers of clairvoyance and the ability to enter trance states at will for hours in his youth. Once, it is said, he stayed under water for ten minutes while in a trance. His parents did not want to encourage these things, so when Akuete entered his twenties he was sent to Paris to study medicine at the Sorbonne.

He studied there for several years, but before he could complete his training, ancestral spirits called him. On one occasion he heard a knock at the door, walked over, and opened it. Outside was a giant snake, the Great Serpent of Africa. The serpent entered the room, threw him on his bed, and then entered him, ending up by becoming a crown on his head. The spirits began appearing and talking to Akuete, making further studies of Western medicine impossible. So, he came home to Lome in Togo and undertook studies with traditional voodoo priests to accept his destiny as a traditional healer.

The first time I met Akuete was at a lecture he gave in San Francisco. He began telling about his history and beliefs, but then he said he would provide a demonstration to prove he was not joking. Voodoo practitioners believe that different spirits can be summoned by special patterns of drumming rhythms, so a drummer with Akuete began a captivating beat. Then his translator, psychologist Danny Slomoff, showed us how to do a spiritual dance step of West Africa, which Danny aptly described as a "funky version of the Chicken."

Akuete told us that he would go into a light trance so as not to disturb anything too much. His eyes took on a distant look, and the several hundred people present now stopped dancing and formed a circle with Akuete in the center. Akuete danced lightly and then looked at a woman. She immediately began shaking and trembling. He pointed at another man and he fell into a trance. In five minutes seven or eight others had begun to shake and tremble. Akuete then stopped and explained that the spirits had chosen these people and that they would soon stop shaking as the spirits purged them of negative energies. They did, and all reported they felt much better.

On another occasion when Akuete entered a trance with a smaller group of people, one woman began wildly throwing herself about the room and had to be restrained. Akuete's interpretation was that she had strayed from her life's true path, and when he took on true spiritual powers, the strength of his spiritual attunement with the truth had entrained with her, forcing her inner conflicts to come out all at once in a desperate attempt to prevent her from recognizing her true path in life.

There are lots of interpretations of why we have ecological problems. Consider the shamanic interpretation that Pulitzer Prize–winning Kiowa author N. Scott Momaday puts forth, that the real root of the ecological crisis is because "our civilization is a spirit-killing entity."[10] Spirits are very important to keeping ecological balance, many people insist. Suspend your judgment for a moment and let's look at what nature spirits are like.

A Taxonomy of Nature Spirits

All around the world there is a belief in the existence of non-material entities that seem to share many common characteristics. These spirits seem to fall into five general categories:

1. *Little People.* In Hawaii the stone platform shrines called *heiaus* are said to have been built by the *menehuene,* tiny humanoid peoples who live within the earth by day but come

out at night. Their counterparts in Europe include fairies, sprites, brownies, and elves and can be found in the ocean, beside springs, on earth at special places, and in forest groves.

2. *Angels.* Angelic spirits originate in the upper realms of consciousness and descend to earth, taking on various forms. Throughout the Bible there are accounts of angels appearing to people in wild places, often giving them important information. They do not come to people on command and appear only rarely. Instead they prefer to work through lower spirits, most sources state.

3. *Demons, Trolls, Jinn, and Other Spirits.* These creatures shift shapes and materialize in this reality, being especially common in wild places, where they live in the ground, waters, and air. The Norwegians speak of the *Huldrafolk* and their music, *Huldraslaat,* which is always in a minor key and mournful. Mountaineers say you learn to play it by "laying your ear to the elf hill." When the *Huldrafolk* come out of the ground, they can interchange forms with trees.

   The Jinn of Persia and Arabia, made famous by the genie of Aladdin's lamp, are recognized in the teachings of Muhammad. The Koran recognizes three types of intelligences under Allah: angels, created from light; jinn, from subtle fire; and man, from the dust of the earth.

   Jinn come in three orders: flyers, walkers, and divers. Supposedly they can be either evil or good. Some of their positive virtues derive from their ability to ascend to the lowest heavens and converse with angels, who give them valuable information about the future. Those that do this have accepted the true faith; the rest are bad and work in close association with fallen angels, whose leader is Iblis, "The Despairer."

4. *Ghost Lights, Fox Fire, and Will-o'-the-wisps.* Virtually every district in England has its own version of the "spook light" or "pixie light." In Germany they are called wandering lights. The French speak of the *feux-follets.* The Italians have the *fuoco fatuo.* The Swedes talk about the "lantern-bearers," who

walk over the heath bogs. In Michigan we used to call them swamp gas or will-o'-the-wisps.

The infamous will-o'-the-wisp is also called the *ignis fatuus,* or "foolish fire." The pumpkins we light up on Halloween are said to represent will-o'-the-wisps. Some very reputable people, including my father, talk about seeing will-o'-the-wisps. He described one he saw one day in a Lake Erie marsh as about the size of a basketball, golden in color, and moving around as if it had a mind of its own. In Texas the Marfa Lights have been seen so commonly, the military is now studying them. Some people insist the flamelike lights reported all around the world on summer evenings are just luminescent marsh gases. Others insist they are manifestations of static electricity, such as Saint Elmo's fire, the bluish-white electrical discharges seen on mountaintops and along masts of sailing ships before storms strike. Others insist they are sentient, ghosts or a special form of natural intelligence that can collect natural energies at will. If only we could train them to help catch poachers and polluters . . .

5. *Humanlike Creatures.* In the Himalayas they call them yeti, or the Abominable Snowmen. Indians of the Pacific Northwest speak with respect of the Sasquatch. Among the Koyukons of Alaska they talk about the "woodsman." Both Linnaeus and Pliny the Elder included apelike humanoids in their taxonomic systems of natural history. The Greco-Roman literature abounds with satyrs, fauns, sylvans, and centaurs— all members of the *callicantyari* tribe.

I list this last category of creatures under the classification of spirits because my shaman friends all agree that they do exist and represent a special class of spirit. Because they can choose to be material or not, one has never been caught, shamans tell me.

If I had not interviewed over sixty people (including an entire school bus full of college students) who have seen, heard, or smelled a Bigfoot, or Sasquatch, with stories nearly identical, I'd leave these big hairy creatures off the list. Typically people first sense something different, a sort of anxious jolt of energy. They then report hearing cries or high-pitched screams. The odor is typically musky. If they see something, it is six to eight feet tall, hairy, long-armed, barrel-chested, and walking upright.

A Freudian psychologist would probably say that these people are having hallucinations, that these creatures are symbolic of the human primal id or libido—the raw animal power in each of us. This is one interpretation, but I have a set of photos of giant footprints with five discernible toes, fourteen inches long and six and a half inches wide, that I took in a dried-up streambed in a remote area of the North Cascades. People with feet that big play tackle for the San Francisco 49ers. Bears' feet are much wider and not at all shaped like these tracks. I have no idea who or what made those tracks, but my Indian friends insist the Bigfoot is more than another sensational story in the tabloids.

Mary Alsup, a psychologist who works on the Trinidad Indian reservation in northern California, Bigfoot country, reports that the Karok tribe say that if you are out in the woods and come upon a Bigfoot, do not be afraid. Look the creature directly in the eye, and like a spark of lightning a jolt of energy will jump between you, and you will acquire the secret wisdom of nature.

LAND AND REVELATION

At one end of the continuum of encounters with nature the person who has them is in control of what is going on. At the other end of the continuum of experiences where nature can be a teacher are revelations that involve total surrender of consciousness, allowing mind and nature to merge into one dynamic whole. According to Vine Deloria, Jr., who has conducted an extensive study of visionary experiences among the Lakota tribe, revelations typically have the following qualities:[11]

1. The person involved is not in control. Something seems to come and grab you, and while you are in its grasp, the world

changes. You can undergo ritual procedures to increase the chances of revelations happening, but you are not the one who decides whether they will take place or what will happen.

2. When the revelation is in progress, the normal qualities of time and space are altered.

3. The person involved is aware of a definite shift in energy and consciousness, which suggests the existence of another dimension of reality.

4. The experience itself is educative, but the content is less personal and more related to other realities, eternal issues, or broader social and cultural matters.

5. Land and place are key to revelations, whereas reflections can happen almost anywhere.

6. Revelations often have a spiritual quality but do not necessarily have anything to do with religion.

7. When a person has a revelation, his or her life may be profoundly changed, with implications for humanity as a whole or at least for communities and larger cultural systems.

Revelations are well known in the lives of Jesus, Buddha, Muhammad, Confucius, and saints of all traditions. Ordinary people can have revelations, too, and when they do, it may be a call to become an environmental advocate. Recall that Gifford Pinchot and Chief Justice William O. Douglas had powerful revelations that moved their conservationist feelings to expand. The following are three examples of the power of nature to change someone's life.

The sign announces THE WORLD'S GREATEST TACKLE SHOP when you turn into the Loch Lomond Marina in San Rafael, California. Nearing the end of the dock, watchful eyes suddenly greet you from all corners. Normally shy and reclusive black-crowned night herons, snowy egrets, and more gulls than you can count are quietly sitting on every available piling, just a foot or two away. They should be in trees or far out in the marsh. What strange spell has tamed them?

Keith Fraser, the owner of the Loch Lomond Live Bait Shop, is a conservationist in the tradition of the Nordic fishermen of Scandinavia, his ancestors. As a kid he grew up along San Francisco Bay, fishing for striped bass and flounders whenever he could. After college he became a teacher and the baseball coach at Terra Linda High School. One afternoon twenty years ago, his life changed because of a fish.

A friend invited Fraser to go fishing out on his boat in the bay. It was rumored there were sturgeon out there—prehistoric monsters with pea-sized brains, no bones, and vacuum-cleaner mouths, some of them twelve feet long. Fraser hooked one and half an hour later was looking eye-to-eye with a seventy-eight-pound living dinosaur.

The way Keith tells it, he caught "sturgeon fever." More and more spare time was used up trying to catch sturgeon number two. Much to his amazement he discovered that at certain times of the year San Francisco Bay fills up with droves of giant sturgeon, but few people catch them without nets. The key to sturgeon success, Fraser discovered, is live bait. As a kid he learned how to dig for ghost shrimp and net grass shrimp. Now it paid off as suddenly he became the most successful sturgeon fisherman in the bay.

News of Fraser's success got out, and people wanted to know his secrets. Soon he began an after-school live-bait business. But the phone kept ringing. Each time he hooked into one of those huge fish (his biggest is 178 pounds, which he released), "sturgeon fever" got worse. Finally he had to quit his job and become a full-time bait-and-tackle-shop operator.

Physically Keith Fraser is a sturgeon-sized man, six feet four inches tall with a booming coach's voice. It seemed as though he had linked with his aquatic archetype and owned his "fisherman medicine," for Fraser became known as Mr. Sturgeon. When Keith Fraser began to share his sturgeon techniques with other people, crowds gathered. One Friday night upward of twelve hundred people crammed into the Corte Madera Recreation

Center to hear Keith's sturgeon wisdom. Police had to turn away over five hundred more because the room was already at nearly twice its capacity. Years later the crowds still keep coming for the sturgeon sermon.

Being out on the bay daily, Fraser could see pollution worsening. The striped bass were disappearing. Something had to be done. In 1980, at his breakfast table, he called together a group of friends, and the United Anglers of California was born. Today UAC represents over seventy thousand Californians and is the largest and most rapidly growing environmental organization in California.

Moved by the slow, persistent, strong spirit of the sturgeon, Fraser's influence has grown. A tackle manufacturer has named a rod after him. Kids ask for his autograph when he gives his sturgeon sermon. Then, in 1989, the sturgeon spirit moved him to become the Bay Area's conservationist version of Batman—"bait man."

"The Army Corps of Engineers was dumping 680,000 cubic yards of dredging spoils a month near Alcatraz Island," Fraser says with a growl. All around the eyes of long, sharp-beaked birds are on him. He reaches down into a tank and tosses a fat minnow to Old One-Eye, a male black-crowned night heron with one eye. The place turns into bedlam, birds everywhere squawking for theirs.

"The water was the color of coffee with cream in it, and the Corps said the junk they were getting out of the most polluted areas of the bay wasn't harming anything," Fraser continues, the birds now seeming like cheerleaders. As most conservationists know, the Army Corps of Engineers is a formidable force. Normal political action was getting nowhere. Fraser got on the phone and started talking. Soon he had a flotilla of 150 boats filled with reporters waiting all around Alcatraz Island. The Corps backed down and stopped dumping, agreeing to "study the problem."

"Today the bay is clearer than it's been in years," Fraser says proudly. Then the phone rings as another order for shrimp comes in. As I stand outside, the birds now look at me, and I remember scenes from Hitchcock's *The Birds.* An eerie feeling sends a chill down my spine. Soon I am inside looking at tackle, buying a lure, a sturgeon amulet with a hook, so that I can safely get back to my car. The birds now seem less ominous. I have made my sacrifice at their shrine to honor their wizard. A night heron lets me feed it. I feel accepted into their circle and decide to sign up to take my son out sturgeon fishing on the bait shop's charter boat, *The Superfish.* Fraser's magic works the next day as we catch five living dinosaurs, the largest weighing sixty-six pounds. This delights Fraser, but he urges us to keep *only* what we will eat and throw back any females with eggs to help save the species.

Across the bay in Berkeley is another man whom the spirit of nature has possessed. On October 4, 1982, engineer Bert Schwarzschild was on vacation in Italy and decided to climb Monte Subasio, the sacred mountain where, over seven hundred years earlier, Saint Francis preached his sermon to the birds.

As he was ascending the mountain, shots rang out in the distance. Soon the trail was littered with hundreds of shotgun shells. "I realized that I had not seen or heard a single bird," Schwarzschild says, "because they were allowing songbird hunting on Saint Francis's mountain."

He continued his climb and decided to spend the night on the mountain. Lying there in his sleeping bag, he could not stop feeling sad and horrified about the killing of birds on the mountain. Suddenly he heard a whirring of wings near his feet. Out of the darkness came the most beautiful bird song he had ever heard. Ornithologists told him that it must have been a nightingale. Like an arrow, the notes shot right through his heart, and he decided that he was going to do something about the killing.

The next day Bert came down off the mountain and began organizing. In a few months he succeeded in mounting a worldwide campaign that moved the government authorities to pass a moratorium on the killing of songbirds on Monte Subasio. Continued persistence resulted in the establishment of a permanent nature reserve and environmental education center, Subasio Regional Park. Bert Schwarzschild has since gone on, in the spirit of Saint Francis, to found the worldwide Assisi Nature Council to promote the teachings of Saint Francis, for, as he says, "If we succeeded in bringing back the songbirds to Assisi, our effort can inspire others elsewhere to make peace with nature."

Poet Michelle Berditschevsky felt drawn to build a home in seclusion on the slopes of Mount Shasta, some two hundred miles north of San Francisco, in hopes of tapping its powerful inspirational force. One day she went out for a walk on the mountain. In the crystal-clear cold mountain air she suddenly heard a voice calling out, "I need your help," a little like the voice in the movie *Field of Dreams*.

The idea of a voice coming from nowhere frightened her, but she sat down and listened. Soon it became apparent that the mountain was talking to her. A few days later the experience took on new light when she discovered that a massive ski resort was being proposed for Shasta and that the area to be developed contained Panther Meadows, a place sacred to Indians of the area that contains a healing spring.

Soon Michelle began talking with others about the ski resort. She found the community deeply divided between the preservationists and the prodevelopers, who saw the ski resort as badly needed for the local economy. Angry words were exchanged at town meetings. Threatening phone calls came into the poet's home. Her allies found their car tires slashed.

One night Berditschevsky sat in her home, afraid, and wondering why this had come to her. In the stillness of the mountain air it dawned on her that as a poet she could be a voice for the spirit of the mountain. Poetry began to flow out of her, and she reports feeling swept along by "an incredible energy that wouldn't let me sleep more than a few hours a night."

Despite strong opposition Michelle and her supporters have

built a strong movement whose allies include the state attorney general. When all this started, she knew next to nothing about environmental-impact statements, resource conservation, and ski resorts. Today she is an expert, blending the emotional eloquence of a poet with her new expertise to stand as a formidable foe to any opponent. She and her allies are seeking to have Mount Shasta declared a World Heritage Site by UNESCO.

SKALALITUDE

In 1989 I took my graduate class in environmental psychology from the California Institute of Integral Studies on a field trip to the Ring Mountain Preserve in Tiburon, California. Ring Mountain is an eastern finger of Mount Tamalpais, which juts out into San Francisco Bay as the backbone of the Tiburon peninsula.

From the standpoint of natural science, Ring Mountain is an important ecological reserve because it is the sole place in the world where the Tiburon mariposa lily grows. Today's hike, however, is a search to perceive the spirit of Ring Mountain, which culminates in a visit to the ancient Miwok Indian fertility stone that sits atop Ring Mountain. Leave your left-brain rational mind in the car. Suspend judgment, and experiment with ways of perception that have been practiced by humans since the Paleolithic age.

As the group gathers at the northern trailhead, I ask them to form a circle. From my backpack I take out a little bag of cornmeal. I take out a pinch and say a prayer. Then I take out a rattle. We stand silently for a few moments, attuning our minds to the place. Then I begin to shake the rattle in accord with the feeling of place. Slowly the energy builds. After a minute or so I begin to whistle a simple refrain that I learned from the Peruvian shaman Don Eduardo Calderon. Around the circle people entrain to the rhythm of the rattle and the melody. A sense of community is building. People's faces seem to become more alive. Now I face the east, continuing the melody. I whistle until the pitch changes to an octave higher. Don Eduardo says this is when the spirit of that direction has joined the circle. I call to all four directions, then the world above and the world below. Then, as if by prior agreement, we all stop at once and stand in the enriched silence for a minute.

Noting the sign to watch for ticks, we pass through the gate and begin our ascent. A hundred yards along the trail a red-shafted flicker comes flapping by, letting out a couple of high-pitched calls. The bird darts like an arrow for a grove of oak trees on a side trail. The spot where the bird lands just happens to be our first stop, a traditional Miwok Indian acorn-grinding stone beside a small stream. The flicker has now become our guide, and rightfully so, for the Miwoks saw the red-shafted flicker as a sacred bird.

At the grinding stone, after people experiment with the mortar and pestle, I ask everyone to be silent and close their eyes. Then as I shake my rattle, I ask them to imagine what it would have been like to be here in this place two hundred years ago. After three or four minutes I stop rattling. One woman reports her awareness of just how much work it had been to turn bitter acorns into edible mush. Several people say historic scenes of the area had come to mind, and they are impressed by how many more trees had once covered the hillside. One person admits to hearing a soft, woman's voice singing in a strange tongue. Acorn Woman is with us.

The group continues up the mountain on a trail beside the brushy banks of the stream. As we move up the mountain, the flicker moves ahead of us, joined by a couple of scrub jays, providing a group escort.

Our next stop is a place where a deer trail comes down to the stream and a small spring emerges from the bank. I talk about the Celtic concept of "track lines" of nourishing earth energies that animals follow, and add that all around the world people say that there are spirits who live where springs surface. I toss a little cornmeal on the ground and chant for a couple of minutes. Most of the group reports feeling a happy feeling or presence about this place. One person says he thinks he hears "tiny bells" in the air, which is what many people say is the sound of "fairy voices."

The flicker now leaves on undulating wing beats. No sooner is our red-shafted guide gone than his replacements appear: two playful ravens. Among many tribes the raven is the creator of the earth. In Europe ravens supposedly guide seekers to the Holy Grail. For sacred places there often seems to be an animal guardian that presides over the place, becoming an embodiment of the spirit of that place. Nearly every time I've come to Ring Mountain, these two ravens seem to meet me. I understand them to be the animal guardians of the mountain.

As we walk up the next quarter mile of trail, the ravens play overhead, squawking loudly in *orc, orc* language. Then, as we come to the spring that is the headwaters of the stream we've followed up the mountain, the ravens land in the rocks ahead of us, as if patiently waiting while we stop for some quiet time. On either side of this spring is a giant tree, each an elder of its species for this place. One is a bay tree, the ceremonial tree of the Miwoks and Pomos, whose pungent leaves are burned in ritual sacrifice. The other is a coast oak, whose acorns were the equivalent of corn for peoples of northern California.

The group sits beside the spring as if it is an altar. I let my mind sink down, down into the ground until I feel a harmonic connection with the root of the spring. Then I pick up the rhythm of the place with the rattle and chant. After a minute or so I become quiet, and we sit in silence for another minute or two. Everyone in the group reports feeling their minds drawn down into the earth at this place to encounter a sense of significant presence. Several people report hearing a deep bass booming voice that seems to be bubbling up out of the ground like the voices of the Ents in Tolkien's hobbit tales. As we sit beside the spring, suddenly from the west a turkey vulture gliding at treetop level passes right over our heads, the bird's shadow bisecting our circle. One girl in the group lets out a startled cry at the bird's sudden appearance so close overhead. Then the ravens begin calling again. We get up and continue to the top, with the two black birds in the lead.

In a matter of minutes we arrive at the Miwok fertility stone on the top—a gray-green, soft, smooth rock with many old circular and semicircular petroglpyhs carved in it. Once Miwok couples would make pilgrimages to this stone to carve these shapes, which resemble the vaginal birth opening. Chanting and praying as they carved, the woman would smear the sacramental rock dust on her body as a prayer to increase fertility and aid childbirth. Today we, too, say prayers at the rock, but more for its protection than anything else, for vandals have ruthlessly chipped away at the old markings and added modern graffiti over ceremonial sacred art. JOHN LOVES MARY somehow captures the spirit of the rock. Anyone who uses a chisel or hammer to hack away at a stone symbol of a vulva has serious sexual problems.

Turning back down the mountain, two hundred yards down the trail, we come upon a herd of seven deer. The number seems fascinating, because there are seven students in the group. At that time, overhead, a red-tailed hawk circles. As we come to the end of the trail, a large hawk-wing feather is lying in the path.

As I say thank you to the mountain, I hear the voice of Acorn Woman saying I should guide more people to this place and have my picture taken beside the stone. Later I arrange for this. No sooner is the picture taken than the *San Francisco Examiner* calls and wants a picture of me. The picture then appears in a special issue.

When the class reconvenes, the woman who had been startled by the vulture that flew over the spring says that as the bird appeared above us, she felt her mind drawn upward, and it seemed as though a "spark" of something jumped between her and the black bird. She says in that instant she saw the vulture to be a part of her and she felt a deeper connection being made with her higher self. She was raised in a very strict manner, which did not encourage individuality. The bird, she says, seemed to symbolize what she must do: accept her own spiritual path and "take flight" to become herself.

Like lightning bugs flashing in the twilight of a warm summer evening, reflective experiences shed new light on life in a way that makes us aware of new facets of ourselves or plays old chords in a new, stronger manner. When revelation comes, mountains are moved, and sometimes saved. Because of our lack of nature kinship, we don't even have a good vocabulary to talk about these things. Among the Salish tribe of the Pacific Northwest, there is a word, *skalalitude,* that describes what life is like when true nature kinship exists. *Skalalitude* means "when people and nature are in perfect harmony, then magic and beauty are everywhere."

NATURE
AS HEALER

*Nature is but another name for health,
and the seasons are but
different states of health.*

—HENRY DAVID THOREAU
Journal, August 23, 1853

Hippocrates, the father of modern medicine, who lived to be 109, counseled that "Nature is the cure of all illness." No one understood the truth of Hippocrates' wisdom more than Theodore Roosevelt, boxer, Rough Rider, naturalist, hunter, mountain climber, and president of the United States from 1901 to 1909.

When you walk into the American Museum of Natural History in New York City, a golden plaque high on the wall to the left preserves Teddy Roosevelt's spirit: "There are no words that can tell the hidden spirit of the wilderness, that can reveal its mystery, its melancholy."

Born in New York City on October 27, 1858, Roosevelt's early education was primarily tutoring, because, in his own words, "I was a sickly, delicate boy, [who] suffered much from asthma." Walks in Central Park helped kindle a fondness for nature, but his lifelong interest in natural history was ignited one day when, walking up Broadway, he came upon a market displaying a dead seal. "That seal filled me with every possible feeling of romance and adventure," Roosevelt exclaimed.[1] He begged his father to get its skull for him. With that seal skull he began his collection of skulls, skeletons, and stuffed skins, which was to become the Roosevelt Museum of Natural History, some of which is still at the Smithsonian Institution.

Teddy's asthma didn't respond well to conventional treatments. Relief finally came when he was sent to the spas of Europe for a "nature cure" followed by an African hunting safari, where Roosevelt is reported to have shot nearly everything in sight. Since some asthmas have psychosomatic roots of suppressed anger, this African trek may have provided a suitable environment for the young Roosevelt to vent his toxic negativity. Forever after, Roosevelt regularly took vacations to health spas, such as Glenwood Springs, Colorado, and/or to adventurous hunting or fishing spots to relieve stress and to regenerate.

"All hunters should be nature-lovers," Roosevelt later wrote. To repay his debt to nature for enabling him to heal his physical and emotional wounds, during his presidency Roosevelt created five national parks (Crater Lake, Wind Cave, Platte, Sully Hill, and Mesa Verde); four wildlife refuges in Oklahoma, Arizona, Montana, and Washington; and fifty-one bird reserves. He also established the buffalo herd in Yellowstone National Park and passed the National Monuments Act.

STYLES OF HEALING

Modern medicine is primarily allopathic in approach. That is, it seeks to cure dis-ease by producing a condition different from or incompatible with the dis-ease. The most common allopathic treatments use chemical drugs to suppress the symptoms of an illness (physical or mental) or to directly attack pathogenic organisms. Attempting to remove the illness or its physical manifestation by means of surgery is also popular. Physical fitness, rest, and relaxation are prescribed for prevention, along with immunizations and overall sanitation. This approach has been especially effective with acute trauma and prevention of public health problems. Allopathy favors studying very small units, such as atoms and molecules, to understand and conquer disease. It arises from the Newtonian-Cartesian mechanical model of science, which says that everything can be best explained by physics and chemistry.

There are three general problems with allopathy. One is that new infectious agents are continually being created that are often resistant to existing chemical strategies. A second is that many physicians perform surgery when it may not be necessary. The third issue is that powerful chemicals often have damaging side effects as bad or worse than the original illness. Some people estimate that as many as 50 percent of all medical patients today are treated for illnesses created by side effects of other medical methods.

In contrast, natural-healing approaches such as homeopathy and naturopathy devote more attention to strengthening the overall homeostatic system of the patient and its ability to ward off dis-ease forces, rather than targeting pathogenic organisms or suppressing symptoms. Some of the common treatment strategies of natural healing include tonics to strengthen organs and systems, cathartics to cleanse the body of toxins, and some homeopathic remedies that intensify symptoms, with the intention of triggering deep biochemical reserves of self-healing. Rest, relaxation, and fitness are also prescribed, as well as organic foods and massage, and there is a strong mental-spiritual component. The healing process is generally slower, but the cure is believed to be much deeper and more long-lasting.

Modern medicine is a potent force for healing, as well as a potential source of dis-ease. Rather than jumping into the debate over which is best when, this chapter seeks to shed light on how nature healing works to help each person take advantage of the natural healing powers Hippocrates spoke of so highly.

. . .

Many people go to the country when they are ill, but not everyone is healed by the experience. Faced with death, some people simply let go and die. Others resist. Psychologist Lawrence LeShan finds three general kinds of attitudes in those who, when confronted with a serious illness, don't want to die. They are: (a) people who fear death and/or the pain associated with death; (b) people who want to live for others (not themselves); and (c) those who want to live because they want to "sing their own song" for the joy and meaning of being themselves.

"For reasons I do not fully understand, the body will not mobilize its resources for either or both of the first two reasons. Only for the third will the self-healing and self-recuperative abilities of the individual come strongly into play."[2]

No one understood and lived the truth of LeShan's research better than Australian track coach Percy Wells Cerutty. In 1938 Percy was a sickly forty-three-year-old government worker, too ill to continue his job. Doctors said he would die in less than a year. Deep down inside of him, Cerutty sensed a fire still glowing despite his weakened body. He retreated to the bush, living off the land, eating raw foods, and learning to walk, run, and exist from the aborigines. Under these conditions his health slowly came back as he followed a regimen that included considerable running and physical exercise. At fifty-one Cerutty ran one hundred miles in twenty-four hours and later won the Victoria Marathon. His raw vitality and brazen spirit attracted athletes, and soon he developed a training camp at Portsea, which was to become the grooming grounds for thirty world-record holders he coached during his career, including Herb Elliott, John Landy, Dave Stephens, and Albert Thomas. "There should be nothing inhibited, regimented, formalized, fixed, or dictated in running," Percy maintained.

Drawing on his observations of the "world's best runners"— children, animals, and aborigines—Cerutty developed running styles like horses', with varied gaits and tempos such as the canter, the gallop, and the surge, which included letting out a bloodcurdling yelp as you passed your opponents. In his seventies he led his students, most of whom were world-class distance runners, on long barefoot runs in the sand dunes. His life's motto written in his fitness book, *Be Fit or Be Damned,* was, "It is not merely that you are alive, but how much alive you are that is important."

During his regeneration period in the bush, Cerutty discovered that raw or slightly cooked foods were the most nutritious. He said this was because they had more "life principle." Cerutty's conclusion about the life force and health is in complete agreement with that of the unorthodox but highly successful natural healer, Edgar Cayce, who said that "healing is allowing the life force to flow through, and its action is to stimulate and arouse each cell of the body to its proper activities."

Cayce's definition of healing may sound esoteric, but looking through the pages of medical-school textbooks, you probably won't find much better. Some references will define health in terms of absence of symptoms of dis-ease, but is that health or maintenance? Health is a dynamic process, maintained by periodic stressing—as when the immune system becomes activated to fight off a cold or one engages in rigorous aerobic exercise. This generates waste products that the body must flush out or they become toxic. Each of us is like a living song played by the forces of nature, with the key to health being the ability to change along with the ever-changing moods of the seasons and the periods of the moon and stars, and dispose of any residual wastes or toxins associated with each cycle of change.

Attitude is a measure of self-esteem, and attitudes do affect the life force. A major health problem among many people today is that they have lost their sense of being able to control their lives. Norman Cousins states, in his classic study of self-healing, *The Anatomy of an Illness as Perceived by the Patient,* that up to 90 percent of all patients who seek medical help are suffering from disorders that are well within the range of their body's self-healing ability.

Archetypes are symbolic representations of the deeper truths of life. When I was in Oregon, I met a living archetype of what the modern mechanical model is doing to people and nature. The client was a full-blooded Native American woman in her late twenties. Her physical symptom was that all the joints on the left side of her body were stiff, sore, and swollen.

The condition began when she was eighteen, she told me, and had gotten progressively worse. She went on to explain that up until she was fifteen she had lived with her family on the reservation, hunting, fishing, and gathering wild foods. She had scars on her arm from a time when she'd killed a deer with a knife.

Her parents had died when she was fifteen, and she was sent to live in a loving but conservative white home in a city. She graduated with honors from high school and went on to do graduate work in college. It seemed that the more "successful" she became, the sicker she got.

Modern research has shown that the left side of the body and the right side of the brain deal primarily with emotions, feelings, and intuitions—the mental functions that she had heavily relied upon when living on the reservation. Moving into the modern world, where rational, analytical, logical thinking dominates and is associated with the right side of the body and the left side of the brain, she had to shut down her emotional-intuitive faculties to conform. Her physical condition was an expression of not only her personal problem but the imbalance of society as a whole.

The therapy she developed, after she came to understand her problem as denial and not just arthritis (which was a symptom), was to first vent her pent-up anger about losing her earlier natural lifestyle. More than one pillow was destroyed, and many logs were split in addition to therapy sessions. She found that a massage or chiropractic adjustment before psychotherapy made her emotions more immediately accessible. To complete her cure, she had to re-create a lifestyle more in tune with the seasons, which meant quitting her job as a research technician and devoting her energies to food gathering and preparation, gardening, and arts and crafts. When she first came to see me, she could hardly walk. A year later she was playing basketball. Her former doctor was fuming because he had diagnosed her as having incurable arthritis and had been treating her with cortisone shots. She was considering suing him for malpractice.

The research of Elmer and Alyce Green at the Menninger Foundation shows that our minds have the capacity to influence many physical conditions that previously were thought to be beyond conscious mental control, including heart behavior, brain rhythms, and many "involuntary" muscles of organs throughout the body. Jack Schwarz, a naturopathic healer from Oregon, for example, has shown that he can choose whether he will bleed or not when a knitting needle pierces his arm. When the needle is withdrawn, the wound shows visible signs of healing within a few hours.

These three examples—Teddy Roosevelt, Percy Wells Cerutty, and the Indian woman—support Karl Marx's view that "estranged labor . . . estranges man's own body from him as it does external nature and his spiritual essence, his human being."[3] All three patients would shortly have died if the course of their illness had not reversed itself. The common pattern of their cures involves letting go of modern society's patterns and demands, immersion in natural settings where schedules can be dropped, and venting negative feelings and allowing intuition to guide one's life into harmony with natural rhythms and instinctual desires while eating a diet of primarily natural, organic foods.

Too often people get the impression that self-healing, like dieting or exercise, is just a matter of finding the right plan to follow. True healing arises from establishing contact with the psychological roots that are the touchstones of your basic identity. This foundation then guides your intuition to search out and establish corresponding harmonic sympathies in the world around us, creating a primal link between nature within and without. This natural harmonic chord then energizes the unique crystalline-structured essence that is the ultimate core of your being, the center-point nucleus of matter-spirit around which all our symbols and energies swarm like planets in a solar system circling a golden sun. Healthy intuition grows from this center point, and an ecological conscience is cultivated as a by-product.

In his penetrating study of natural healing, *The Body Electric,* physician Robert Becker reflects, "Our search for the healing power isn't so much an exploration as an act of remembering something that was once intuitively ours, a form of recall in which the knowledge is passed on or awakened by initiation and apprenticeship to the man or woman of power. . . . All worthwhile medical research and every medicine man's intuition is part of the same quest for knowledge of the same elusive healing energy."[4]

Each person is his or her own ultimate nature healer, and each process of healing is unique. Some people, like Percy Cerutty, are able to make the journey by themselves. Others need guidance and help from those who have made the journey already. In the following section we will look at healers skilled at working with natural forces. Life results from elements—earth, air, water, and fire—that come together to create wholeness. Techniques must be mastered, but the best healers have a special calling to work with natural elements in a unique way, their "medicine," Indians call it. Their methods are an expression of their nature kinship; nature healers work with allies more than with antibodies.

HEALING WITH NATURAL ELEMENTS

WATER

When Carolus Linnaeus journeyed to Lapland in 1732, he noted in his journal, *A Tour of Lapland,* that "The Laplanders treasure snow water as if it were the choicest wine." At first the physician was skeptical, but then he began drinking snowmelt and became a convert, proclaiming, "I am persuaded that those who could undertake a journey to the alpine country would derive full as much benefit from coming hither to drink snow water, as from frequenting mineral springs."

Water is "the primary organ of rhythm, the heart of nature, the element in which we can discern nature's heartbeat," conclude Theodor and Wolfram Schwenk in their masterful study of the science and spirit of water, *Water: The Element of Life.* But if you turn on the tap, do you get "live water" or "dead water," they ask?

To drive home their point that live water, which is directly taken from nature in a pristine state, differs from dead water, which may be chemically acceptable but without vital force, the Schwenks have developed a unique, revealing test. They take pictures at a very fast speed as drops of water fall onto a clear glass lens, and these drops form patterns that are striking signatures of the nature of the water's quality and origins. Live water from snowmelt or a spring produces beautiful rosette patterns, like the mandalas meditators perceive to be the pure sounds of the universe. Water from a heavily polluted stream yields flattened shapes with much smaller, less developed patterns.

The aesthetic results of the Drop-Picture Method test lend support to studies in Russia by Vadim and Igor Zelepukhin of the Institute of Fruit-Growing and Vine-Growing in Kazakhstan. In one study they cut plant leaves and placed them in tap water, boiled water, or fresh snowmelt for an hour and then reweighed them to determine water absorption. Typically the leaves in snowmelt absorbed two to three times as much water as the leaves in the other waters.

In another study they soaked seeds in the three types of waters and then planted the seeds. Cotton seeds that had been soaked in snowmelt grew plants that yielded 10 to 12 percent more cotton than normal. The same superiority of yield was found to be true for tomato, potato, maize, and wheat seeds. "The experimental plants were superior to the control plants in all physiological characteristics," the Zelepukhins found. When they gave the same "magic water" to animals, they also recorded measurable positive differences, such as a rise in blood hemoglobin, great vitality, and faster weight gain.[5]

"Water can be made into a medicine," says Rolling Thunder. His approach is to fill a clean glass jar with spring water, place it where the sun's rays first strike it in the morning, and pray over it. Drinking water he has doctored this way seems to taste sweeter and, to me, feels softer.

Water also seems to have a memory. Ambrose Worrall, an engineer and husband of the famous spiritual healer Rev. Olga Worrall, found that when certain people place their hands beside but not touching glass containers of water and pray over them, the surface tension of the water changes. He believed this change in surface tension is an indication of a person's calling to be a spiritual healer and proposed a measurement system to describe this healing power, with the unit of measurement being the "Worrall":[6]

$$Worrall = \frac{initial\ surface\ tension - final\ surface\ tension}{10}$$

Water from the holy well at Saint Breward in Cornwall is supposed to cure sore eyes. Beside or under many of the great cathedrals of Europe, including Chartres, Nîmes, and Glastonbury, there are similar sacred springs. More than four million pilgrims—including sixty thousand sick people—annually make pilgrimages to Our Lady of Lourdes in France to drink and bathe in the spring water from the grotto where Saint Bernadette, at age fourteen, reported seeing the Virgin Mary eighteen times. There are many documented healings attributed to these springs and others, but when Ambrose Worrall analyzed a sample of water from the spring at Lourdes, he could find nothing unusual about the water chemistry that could account for its healing powers. This is not true, however, of all natural springs.

Hippocrates, Aristotle, Homer, and Herodotus were all early advocates of springs for healing, such as those at Thermopylae, which have been used medicinally for over twenty centuries. King Herod frequented thermal baths at Calirrhoe, near the Dead Sea. Shamans all around the world consider certain springs to be some of the most potent allies.

On April 20, 1889, Dr. Winslow Anderson won the Annual Prize of the Medical Society of the State of California for his essay *Mineral Springs and Health Resorts of the State of California with a Complete Chemical Analysis of Every Important Mineral Water in the World.* He was inspired by the famous healing spas of Europe and the Middle East, such as Wiesbaden and Baden-Baden in Germany, Montecatini-Terme in Italy, Warmbad Villach in Austria, and Haméi Zohar in Israel, as well as ancient Rome, where mineral waters were almost the only medicines used for over five centuries, and the springs at Thermopylae, which have been in active use for health for over two thousand years.

He visited most of the over two hundred then known cold and hot mineral springs of California and found them effective for treating many chronic articular disorders, rheumatism, synovitis, gout, indigestion, dyspepsia, torpidity of the liver and intestinal tract, glandular enlargement, renal affections, Bright's disease, irritation and inflammation of the bladder, brickdust deposit, calculus or stone in the bladder, diabetes, blood glandular diseases, scrofula, syphilitic cutaneous contaminations, and others.

Anderson also issued a warning that although mineral waters, taken internally or bathed in, may appear bland and harmless, they are potent therapeutic agents that can accomplish much good when used properly but can also be very harmful, even fatal, when not used properly.

The healing properties of mineral springs are realized by drinking the waters, bathing in the waters, immersing oneself in their muds, sitting on the stones in the springs (which may carry electromagnetic energies), and applying the mosses and algaes that grow in the spring waters to the skin. Immersion in water can heal through temperature (which affects the muscles and nervous system), osmosis through the skin's semipermeable membrane, and electrolytic exchange. The following table is a brief listing of Anderson's findings for natural springs in California, according to their chemistry:

TABLE 6-1
HEALING PROPERTIES OF NATURAL MINERAL SPRINGS
ACCORDING TO WINSLOW ANDERSON

1. *Acidic Mineral Springs.* Springs have been found to contain significant amounts of sulphuric, hydrochloric, and nitric acids, and nearly all contain some dissolved carbonic-acid gas. Some acidic waters can be very helpful to people with poor digestion, chronic lead poisoning (sulfuric acid springs), bladder cysts, fevers, chronic liver troubles, and certain skin diseases.

2. *Alkaline Springs.* May be naturally carbonated like so many of the commercially available spring waters on the market today, but generally have a great deal more dissolved solids than anything you'll find on a supermarket shelf. Our family well in Michigan is an alkaline spring that has been successfully used by some people for acid-stomach troubles, rheumatism, chronic constipation, diabetes, and kidney problems.

3. *Alum Springs.* Not much value, except perhaps for hemorrhaging and uterine douches.

4. *Arsenical Springs.* Anderson suggests that "small draughts should be taken half an hour before meals" from springs with traces of arsenic for irritative dyspepsia, chronic gastric catarrh, gastralagia, and enteralgia.

5. *Borax Springs.* Can be useful for sore throats.

6. *Bromine and Bromide Springs.* Doctors of Anderson's era

prescribed bromine-rich waters for rheumatism, gout, blood diseases, goiter, synovitis, and so forth, as well as mental stress, skin diseases, and syphilitic swellings.

7. Calcareous or Earthy Mineral Waters. Waters with considerable calcium, carbonate, and sulfate—"hard" waters—tend not to be very useful, except perhaps for rickets and osteoporosis.

8. Carbonated Mineral Springs. Waters rich in carbonates, bicarbonates, soda, lime, potash, magnesium, and so on, can be used like sodium bicarbonate and associated drugstore medicinals.

9. Chalybeate or Ferruginous Springs. Waters with high concentrations of iron salts can be very useful for anemia and other blood diseases.

10. Chlorinated or Muriated Springs. Naturally chlorinated waters can be very helpful for gout, scrofula, and abdominal problems, as well as chronic catarrh and rheumatism.

11. Iodine Mineral Springs. These waters have great therapeutic value for a wide range of conditions including goiter, enlargement of internal organs, chronic bronchitis, pleurisy, chronic malaria, and asthma.

12. Magnesium Springs. "Bitter waters," as magnesium springs are called, can be very helpful as a laxative, as anyone who has ever taken epsom salts can attest. Headaches, acid stomach, and flatulence can also be aided by magnesium springs.

13. Siliceous Springs. Not generally used for medicine. Immerse some wood in one of these springs for a few days and it becomes petrified.

14. Sulphurous Mineral Springs. The "rotten eggs" smell of a sulfur spring alerts you to its presence often long before you see the water. Rheumatism, gout, and skin diseases respond to sulfur springs.

. . .

There are healing springs in every state and country around the world. Soap Lake in central Washington State, or *Smokiam*, which means "healing waters" in the tongue of the local Indians, contains more than sixteen minerals known to be associated with healing. The waters are so rich in dissolved solids that on a windy day piles of foam build up along the shores. If you let the water evaporate, bath salts will form. Some people collect and sell these crystals, so you can have a Soap Lake in your bathtub.

Another site of healing waters is Indian Hot Springs, a group of twenty-two artesian springs in rugged Hudspeth County right along the dusty banks of the Rio Grande in West Texas. When Captain Jeff Maltby explored the desert of the northern Rio Grande region in Texas in 1880, he reported in his book *Captain Jeff, or Frontier Life in Texas with the Texas Rangers*, "The old signs and trails leading into the springs indicated that the Indians held the virtues of these springs as the people of old Biblical times held the Pool of Siloam" (a well-known spring just outside of Jerusalem).

In 1952 Jewel Babb and her family bought Indian Hot Springs in the hope of turning it into a profitable resort. Located miles from any human activity and accessible only by a thirty-one-mile-long rough dirt road, the resort never prospered, but poor Mexicans from across the Rio Grande came seeking healing. With them came a folk healer, or *curandera*, named Venezuela, and Mrs. Babb became her student out of necessity. In Mrs. Babb's own words,

> Every time an old timer came to bathe or if I heard of someone knowing something about the springs, I'd go and find them and ask them what they knew about the place. Of course they'd tell me about the many sick people that they'd seen there and many more things. I made it a point to check everything about the place. Why was each water different? Why was one mud black, another grey, pinkish, or white? Why was one water hot, another warm?

All this went on for seven years. There was many healings. And when I finally had to leave the springs, I came away with part or most of the spring's healing power in my mind and hands.[7]

Jewel Babb's life and learning at Indian Hot Springs have been beautifully described by folklorist-writer Pat Ellis Taylor in her book *Border Healing Woman*. As part of her research to understand the spirit of Indian Hot Springs, Taylor went to Indian Hot Springs for a treatment and followed a twenty-one-day regimen spelled out by Mrs. Babb.

The springs are a like a medicine chest; each one's water, muds, and mosses are different, Mrs. Babb explained. The beginning of the cure is the purge, to leach all the tension and toxins from your body. Purging begins with two baths a day, one in the morning and one in the evening, and abstaining from eating any solid food for at least a week. During this time one should drink six to eight glasses of water daily from the Chief Spring.

By the third day Taylor began to feel weak. Although the spring water wasn't extremely hot, she began to notice that as she crawled out of the water after a bath, her heart would be pounding as if she'd been in a scorching steam bath. Each day she would sleep more. Waves of nausea swept through her, and worries would bubble up to consciousness, just like the waters of the spring coming to the surface.

Taylor feels that the purging was accomplished by the strong alkaline chemistry of the Chief Spring. At the end of the first week she felt drawn to eat citrus fruits to restore the acid-base balance of her body, and her discomforts began to subside.

Stripped of some of her tensions, she then went on to bathe in other springs, discovering that each one would affect her differently. At the Sundance Pool she found herself reflecting about oracles living at springs and she had strange, vivid dreams instructing her to drink the water in a certain way. At the Squaw

Spring she and her companions covered their bodies with mud and were delighted at how it softened their skin.

Taylor's twenty-one-day cure ended at the Dynamite Spring. In her account she describes how she felt after her watery death-and-rebirth ordeal:

> When the sun had set and a good portion of the sky had turned colors, I went for my last bath in the Dynamite Spring. Its surface was covered with foam and moss, which I scraped off with a stick so that I could at least see the water I was getting into. Small black birds were racing and skimming over my head, then swooping over the standing water just west of the spring. I felt like a baby, sitting in the pool, rocking in the soft moss; I wondered if any baby could be born in just 21 days; it seemed like it must take more time than that to be ready to come out, be expelled. I remembered an old Bible story about Laman, who was directed to dip himself in the river Jordan to be healed. So I dunked my own head once down completely into the water, then again. The fifth time I held up my arms and the centers of my hands began throbbing in the same way my heart and stomach and temples had taken turns thumping at different times from this pool. The sixth time I threw back my head and held my face up to the sky, which was darkening blue. The seventh time, and I was out of the water. I sat on a stone and let the water dry with the breezes on my skin.[8]

Taylor reports that following this cure she experienced an outflowing of creativity in poems and writing that propelled her into a new level of success as a writer and artist.

EARTH

Every year around Easter time thousands of people make pilgrimages to the "Lourdes of America," Santuario de Chimayó, near Espanola, New Mexico, some of them carrying crosses on their backs. The church is located on the site of an ancient Indian healing spring. Entering the church, people pay their respects to the Catholic icons, but then go on to a small side chamber that contains two astonishing things. One is an enormous pile of crutches. The other is a hole in the floor that exposes the bare earth, which is said to have a miraculous healing power. To get the benefits of the soil, people reach down and collect a little to take home with them. I know some very scientific people who have little containers of soil from Chimayó in their homes.

At Gurney's International Health and Beauty Spa in Montauk, New York, mud from the Montecatini-Terme spa in Italy is flown in for special mud baths, which are said to soothe sore muscles and soften the skin. Cosmetics giant Revlon also imports Montecatini-Terme mud because the minerals supposedly work miracles on tired skin. Other salons and spas in the United States import mud from Hungary, special places in the American West, and the Dead Sea in Israel, believing that each mud has a different therapeutic value. Some mud potions sell for thirty dollars for a twenty-ounce jar at Macy's in San Francisco.

One of the more famous proponents of taking mud baths was the late religious historian Mircea Eliade. Born in Bucharest in 1907, Eliade reports in his *Autobiography* how his father was afraid of contracting scrofula and took the whole family for the mud baths at Tekirghiol in Romania, ultimately buying a simple cabin there to use when visiting the baths. These healing muds had been known to the Tartars for centuries. Eliade describes their healing process: initially tiring a person "to the marrow" when bathing in the mud, which forces them to rest; but afterward, the bathers become stronger and healthier.

When Mormon pioneer Sam Brannan first visited the simple hotel beside some natural hot springs in southern Sonoma County, California, in 1867, he was immediately taken by the springs, which the local Wappo Indians called *Coo-lay-no-maoch,* or "the oven place." Brannan soon purchased the hotel, named the place Calistoga, and began building a resort, which became an overnight success. One of the guests was writer Robert Louis Stevenson, who, during his honeymoon at the springs in 1880, wrote in his novel *Silverado Squatters,* "The whole neighborhood of Mount Saint Helena is full of sulfur and boiling springs . . . and Calistoga itself seems to repose on a mere film above a boiling, subterranean lake."

Today the town of Calistoga has half a dozen spas offering a variety of hot water baths, massage, and chiropractic treatments. The ultimate treatment, however, is the mud bath, which involves immersing yourself in a tub of a 101–104-degree mixture of volcanic ash, clay, peat moss, and hot mineral water for ten to twelve minutes. Afterward, people will typically shower off the mud and then have a massage or go for a gentle swim. The people in Calistoga are reluctant to make any claims about the healing values of their mud baths, but the lines of people waiting to be immersed in a tub of their mud speak for themselves.

METAL

The new-age movement provides us with many new potentialities, and a few humorous explorations of natural health and healing. In Santa Fe, New Mexico, in 1989, a new-age nonalcoholic bar opened up with "intoxicating" beverages "charged with energies from crystals." The club stayed open about six weeks.

These days it's in vogue to wear crystals. Psychologically speaking, the crystal symbolizes a center point of consciousness and the true self, as well as the mystical "third eye" that lies in the brow and serves to guide people on their spiritual paths.

Native Americans have long cherished crystals, according to Native American clinical psychologist Leslie Gray of San Francisco. "The bones of our ancestors," as Dr. Gray calls crystals, are felt by Indians to possess special powers for channeling healing energies, divining the future, and extracting negative energies from people.

Crystals manifest these abilities most strongly, Gray believes, when they have been treated according to ancient traditions. In Indian cultures, Gray says, power crystals are kept covered at all times, unless they are being used in a ritual setting. This is done to prevent the crystals from becoming contaminated with unwanted energies.

To activate crystals, many tribes use special ceremonies to charge them with natural energies. Commonly this begins with washing the crystal in water from a special spring, then exposing it to a special energy so that it picks up these vibrations, for example leaving one in a forked stick overnight during a solstice or equinox with the point of the crystal aimed at the moon, or striking the crystal on a rock in the ocean between waves.

Other natural metals used for healing include copper and uranium. Copper influences electromagnetic fields, so wearing copper bracelets to help sore joints may actually have an influence by ever so slightly altering the electrical fields of the body, the way an acupuncture treatment does. Many natural healers believe that a serious source of stress for some people who frequent cities is the buildup of static electricity in their bodies, in part due to loss of direct contact with the earth because of the prevalence of concrete, asphalt, and so on, as well as having to live and work with one's feet far above the earth. Some sensitive people feel that copper bracelets help. Aside from the power of suggestion, benefits might be derived from any field effects produced by the copper. Many Indian tribes saw pure copper as a spiritual mineral, capable of manifesting great healing powers. Whenever you find folklore like this which is consistent among numerous cultures, there is almost always a grain of truth modern science can agree with.

Uranium, potentially the most lethal substance on earth, has several uses in natural healing. Natural uranium ore discharges negative air ions as it decays, enlivening the air above uranium ore deposits. Since an abundance of negative air ions is often associated with sacred places, and a number of sacred places of the world are the sites of uranium ore deposits, it's not hard to understand why the Pueblo tribes of the Southwest decry the mining of uranium, saying that it takes the natural healing power of fire from the ground and turns it into destructive powers to terrorize people.

One of the treatments at Indian Hot Springs that the *curanderas* taught Mrs. Babb to use for women with menstrual problems was to sit on uranium-rich rocks in the springs. While Edgar Cayce never visited Indian Hot Springs, he did agree with Jewel Babb that uranium is a healing metal that belongs only in its natural state.

AIR

Air is something we cannot see directly, but we know its presence when a cool breeze passes over our faces while we walk beside the ocean, when the pungent scent of a pine forest intoxicates us, when a flock of geese pass by overhead, and when radiant heat waves cause watery mirages on a hot, dry summer day. Like the rising and falling of the tides, our lungs fill and empty with air twenty-four hours a day—otherwise we die. Air is something we take for granted, unless it becomes polluted, yet air can be a healing force, too.

A breath of fresh air can work wonders if you've been cooped up in a stuffy room. A week by the ocean or at a mountain retreat can do even more, providing you can fully take advantage of the power of breath. With each breath cycle, new oxygen-rich air enters the lungs and carbon dioxide–laden air leaves. On the inhalation the sympathetic nervous system is activated. Exhalation employs the parasympathetic. Some healers say they can know a person's whole life pattern just by watching him or her breathe. Someone who is continually puffing up his chest and never relaxing fully on the exhale is an overachiever, possibly a Type-A person prone to heart problems. Someone who doesn't inhale fully often feels depressed, as if she is always fighting an uphill battle.

The sages of India and the Middle East assert that if you can gain control over your breath, you can gain control over your life. Breathing patterns can be changed. As a first step try the following:

> Take your pulse for fifteen seconds. Record the reading. Now inhale slowly to an eight-count. Hold your breath for an eight-count, and then exhale, slowly, for a sixteen-count. Repeat this half a dozen or more times. Now take your pulse for fifteen seconds. Most people find this slows the pulse down considerably.

If you can master this level of internal control over your breathing, you will most likely find your stress level dropping. A good deep breath of fresh air is often the best thing you can do for yourself in a difficult situation. Making a noise on the exhalation lets off more tension. Some people find that when they combine controlled breathing with visualization, their stress levels drop even more.

> Return to your awareness of breathing. Stand and face the sun if there is daylight. If it is night, imagine the sun's presence in the sky and face in an eastern direction. Raise your hands above your head, palms upward and elbows out. As you inhale, imagine that light is coming through your palms and the center of your forehead and streaming down to your feet. As you exhale, visualize this radiant golden energy rising in spirals and filling your body. Do this nine times. This is an ancient Buddhist healing exercise called the Sunshine Buddha, as taught by Grand Master of Black Tantric Buddhism for the World, Master Thomas Yun Lin (whose work will be described more in the next chapter).

A modern therapy system, holotropic breathing, developed by Stanislav and Christina Grof, employs hyperventilation to help people work through emotional problems and explore new dimensions of consciousness. A typical session of holotropic breathing involves a group of people pairing off, with one person being a breather, the other a helper. In a semidarkened room a carefully selected sequence of music is played as the breathers breathe deeply until hyperventilation occurs. As the breathers lie in a prone position, the charge of excitement built up in the body then pulses around. Mental-emotional blocks manifest as chronic muscle tension. The force of the energy built up through the breathing is often sufficiently strong to overcome these tensions, which have been kept from consciousness. Other times the tension intensifies and has to be massaged to allow new life force to fill the previously chronically tense area. As these areas open up, the material locked in the chronically tense muscles becomes conscious, revealing old traumatic memories and new frontiers of perception and knowledge. The extra energy may also push people into transcendent states of ecstasy, which the Grofs feel have a very important curative value for people, enabling them to go through an ego death and rebirth. Following the breathing session, participants are encouraged to draw mandalas and dance to express their discoveries and integrate the material unearthed. *(This is not a technique recommended for people to try without experienced practitioners, for hyperventilation can lead to apnea and other difficult mind-body states.)*

To a Chinese healer, air contains *chi,* which includes spirit. The same is true of the Hindu concept of *prana,* which is breathed in with the breath. The Pomo Indian *weya* and the Sufi life-force *baraka* seem to be similar concepts.

Modern science and psychology have difficulty understanding how spirit can be associated with air, which they describe in terms of physics and chemistry. When one breathes deeply for a time, hyperventilation occurs. Hyperventilating leads to altered states of consciousness, enabling transpersonal exploration. Air and spirit work together, yet as Norman Cousins pointed out, "the life-force may be the least understood force on earth.[9]

ENVIRONMENTAL FIELDS

The earth's natural electromagnetic field has a normally positive polarity that ranges from near zero to many thousands of volts in the immediate vicinity of a thunderstorm. Inside metal-framed buildings, automobiles, airplanes, and any structure surrounded by metal, the normally changing earth field is zero polarity, creating what is called a Faraday cage. Nearly all plastics, such as those commonly used in clothing, interior design, auto interiors, and for structural materials, have a strong negative charge. All conditions other than the normal natural positive earth field can cause dis-ease in some people, including fatigue, irritability, dizziness, difficulty concentrating, and hypersensitivity to allergic reactions. These conditions may cause discomfort and require the person to work harder to focus on the tasks at hand. In the long run, field disruption may result in weakening of the immune system and allergic reactions.

When she was alive, Frances Nixon, of tiny Thetis Island, which lies to the east of Vancouver Island, in Juan de Fuca Strait in British Columbia, was the most sensitive person I've ever met. You could blindfold Fran and lead her into a room and she would tell you where all the electric outlets were located with near 100 percent accuracy. Then she'd tell you what the carpet was made of, if the appliances in the room were on or off (when no sound was audible from them to the average ear), and for good measure she'd tell you within fifteen minutes when the next high tide would be. As a result of spending many hours alone in nature observing how animals behaved as well as how she felt under various conditions, Fran, an artist by training, developed a way of using her entire body as an instrument for sensing. She discovered that feelings in various parts of the body indicate solar flares, tidal action, magnetic storms, and impending weather-front changes.

To harness this sensitivity for health, Fran developed the Vivaxis Energy System, which is based on staying in harmony with your place of birth. This theory says that during the time we are in the womb, our forming bones and tissues take on an energy imprint of the environmental fields in the area where we are born. Forever after, Fran taught, we are harmonically linked with our place of birth, regardless of where we are on earth. This harmonic connection helps establish personal identity and empowers you to be who you are. We can lose touch with our Vivaxis through accidents, illness, drugs, chemicals, and noxious electromagnetic fields in the surrounding environment. (Check the appendix of this book for information about how to learn more about the Vivaxis System.)

Studies with honeybees, fish, pigeons, sharks, plants, and bacteria have clearly demonstrated how life orients to the earth's electromagnetic fields. Increasingly, scientific data are showing that Fran Nixon's perceptions are accurate readings of natural-field phenomena. If you are a field-sensitive person, Dr. Robert Becker's book *The Body Electric: Electromagnetism and the Foundation of Life* is essential reading. A physician with a lifetime of research on how fields influence health and healing, Becker concludes that proper use of electrical fields may help healing, but exposure to some fields may lead to cancer, mental illness, and other diseases. The World Research Foundation, a leader in research on cross-cultural healing, reports that a study of 500,000 persons regularly exposed to strong electromagnetic fields in Washington State found that 60 percent had a higher rate of leukemia and 75 percent had a higher rate of lymph-gland cancer than a control group.[10]

In Los Angeles there is a radio station that is supposedly so strong that even water pipes carry its vibes. One result of this is that you can hear a concert when you use the bathroom. Humorous but troubling, considering Robert Becker's finding that long-term exposure to human-created fields seems to weaken the body's natural immune system, thus paving the way for people to become sick more easily. The recent invention of personal, inexpensive electromagnetic-field detectors may soon turn us into a legion of field detectives.

Fran Nixon recommended taking frequent baths in baking soda and sea salt and walking barefoot on a sandy beach to neutralize static-energy accumulations. Even if you aren't extremely sensitive, this is good medicine.

PLACE

Among the members of the Maria Lionza religion of Venezuela, the most appropriate place to perform a healing ceremony is at the sacred mountain, Sorté, some three hundred miles from Caracas. Amid the rushing streams and dense tropical foliage on the mountain, many groups come to conduct healing rituals. After a ritual, patients are often instructed to lie on the ground in a certain place to allow the natural energies of the earth to help absorb negative energies and recharge them with fresh, clean life force. Ceremonies at Sorté get better results than any place else for the Maria Lionza followers.

Modern psychology is unable to explain why healings occur so often at Sorté, Lourdes, or Chimayó, but using the outdoors to aid healing has a history even within the modern medical model. "Tent therapy" was used over one hundred years ago by American mental health practitioners, who found that some people recovered from mental dis-ease more quickly in the outdoors. In more recent times Japanese psychotherapists have found that when they took chronic schizophrenics on hiking and camping trips in the country, 80 percent of the patients experienced a remission of symptoms, and improved social and interpersonal relationships.[11] Similar positive results have been found for programs for emotionally disturbed adolescents and senior citizens.

Psychologist Tom Pinkson of Marin County, California, has found that nature has a powerful therapeutic value for helping drug addicts kick their habits. Heroin addicts suffer from low self-esteem and difficulty controlling impulses; the numbing power of the heroin seems to ease their anxiety and give them a fleeting sense of relaxation and euphoria. They lack what Jacob Needleman has called a "first-hand sense of identity."

Working with groups of no more than ten people, Pinkson's program begins with a series of initial meetings to teach basic survival skills as well as some day hikes to acquaint his clients with the outdoors. Many addicts, he finds, have never gone very far from a concrete, steel, and plastic world. Walking in the woods, many discover both new sensory experiences and a whole host of fears that they had been avoiding.

These preparations lead up to three- to seven-day wilderness outings, which include white-water rafting, mountain climbing, and desert hiking, as well as a twenty-four-hour solo with no food or fire. Over several years Pinkson took out over three hundred people, all with self-destructive behavioral problems, and had no accidents. In a follow-up study with thirty-nine people he could locate one year after their outing, 43 percent had made significant lifestyle and behavioral changes that were apparently permanent, while 35 percent had regressed or were incarcerated. This is a much higher recovery rate than normal for hard-core heroin addicts, who are among the most difficult of all drug addicts to work with.

Inspired by his success with heroin addicts, Pinkson has designed a special wilderness experience that includes a pilgrimage to a sacred place and a forty-eight-hour solo. Among his clients who have benefited from this spiritual search for self in nature are businessmen, ex-convicts, priests, and cocaine addicts. Recently one of his clients was a sixty-six-year-old overweight retired college professor who had tested positive for HIV, the forerunner of AIDS. Pinkson guided his puffing client up to an 11,000-foot-elevation pass in the high Sierras for a solo in a snowfield. The professor later reported that during his time alone, trees and rocks spoke to him. A year later, his immune system seems to have strengthened and he has more vitality, energy, and strength, as well as having made a number of positive personality changes toward fuller use of his life and talents.

HERBS

In earlier times herbal medicines were prescribed according to a theory known as the doctrine of signatures. This ancient belief holds that the form and shape of a drug determines its healing value: Walnuts look like brains, so they must be good for the brain; the European species of saxifrage have granular bulblets on their roots, so they must be good for dissolving urinary concretions. This same principle of similarities is one of the reasons why some people believe that deer antlers or rhinoceros horn is good for increasing male sexual potency.

"Herbs have two ways of working. One is by their chemistry, and the other is by their spirit," Dr. John Christopher told me one day during a week-long workshop I produced for him in 1976. A short, stocky man with a wild head of white wavy hair, Dr. John was the living essence of a wizard. In the true spirit of naturopathy he believed that healing always works best when the medicines used trigger the patient's own immune system, which in turn both promotes the natural healing powers of the body and drives out the toxins that are causing the problem. Typically he would begin treatment by placing people on a "cleansing fast" of fruit juice and special herbal tonics to "purify the blood and drive out toxins." During one of his cleansing programs I found a variety of tastes manifesting in my mouth, such as saltiness, sweetness, and bitterness. Dr. John explained calmly that this was my body releasing excess residues from improper eating in the past. As he predicted, after a few days the foul tastes went away, and in addition to feeling rejuvenated, I discovered a new awareness of taste.

Once your system was cleansed, then Dr. John would prescribe herbal remedies to adjust your inner chemistry and activate your body's natural homeostatic healing mechanisms. One time he prescribed the herb gotu kola for me. I began taking it, and in a few days I had a real bout with diarrhea and vomiting. Dr. John simply said that this was my body throwing off toxins. After the purge subsided, I felt a great deal more relaxed. Some of his remedies, such as a daily tonic of a heaping tablespoon of cayenne powder mixed with spring water, would make your hair stand on end, but they worked, and that's what is important in the final analysis.

Privately, John Christopher admitted that some of his best remedies ultimately came from dreams, visions, and conversations with plants. When you meet up with a plant person in the spirit world, the plant becomes an ally, not just an herbal potion. Once a healer gains a plant ally, the potency of the results comes from both the chemical reactions and the sympathetic alignments between the mind of the patient, the healer's mind, and the next world. This is why nature healers speak so fondly of some of their herbs, for they become more like helping assistants than just chemical remedies.

ANIMALS

In Mexico it's rumored that you can cure a child's asthma by putting a chihuahua dog in bed with him. The high rate of respiration of the dog generates a local environmental field that has a strong positive charge that apparently has healing virtues, according to aerospace engineer James Beal. Animals as pets can provide companionship for people, which in itself can be healing, for all too often the letters I.L.L. are really short for "I lack love."

Anthropologist Michael Harner reports in his popular book *The Way of the Shaman* that animal symbols can also have a powerful healing force. Drawing upon years of field research with shamans all around the world, Harner has developed some simple, extremely powerful guided journeys that people use to find "power animals." Upon meeting these numinous animals in the lower world, they then bring these creatures back from the imaginary realm and integrate them psychologically into their waking self, often with very powerful positive results. Shamans say that people become ill when they lose their power, creating holes in their consciousness, Harner explains. These journeys to find their personal totemic power animals seem to fill people up with new energy and meaning, which tap new levels of the body's reserves to fight off illness.

Harner's research is supported by the work of clinical psychologist Jean Achterberg, who uses creative imagery to help people energize their immune system to fight cancer.[12] Working with a woman with lung cancer, Achterberg reports how the woman's cancer went into remission as she was able to befriend a leopard that appeared in her imagery and dreams. The leopard had terrified her for years, but now as she came to feel closeness with the animal, her personal stress level dropped and her cancer symptoms vanished. There is a connection between the leopard within and the leopard without.

FIRE

Another of those people who has special expertise in linking mind and nature to bring about healing is Brooke Medicine Eagle, the great-grandniece of the renowned holy man of the Nez Percé tribe, Chief Joseph.

Trained in both modern humanistic and transpersonal psychology and traditional shamanism, today Brooke runs a retreat center in rural Montana where people burned out by modern society come to regenerate. "The problem of most people today is that they are not embodied," Brooke asserts. "They are taught that God and heaven are someplace else and that their bodies are machines to earn money."

Brooke guides her students through purification processes, including fasting and special diets, prior to the traditional sweat-lodge ceremony. The lodge is a dome-shaped hut constructed in a special, quiet place. A fire is built nearby, and volcanic and metamorphic rocks are placed in the fire to heat up until they glow cherry red. (Sedimentary rocks absorb water, so if you heat them, the water expands into steam and they explode.)

The hot rocks are placed inside the lodge and the door is closed to trap the heat. Outside, the participants strip down and are smudged with the smoke of sweet sage, an herb of purification. Entering into the dark hut is like walking into an oven—a blast of fiery heat sears your sinuses. The participants crouch down in a circle around the rocks. The leader tosses some sage on the rocks and then some water. Clouds of steam billow up into air. Prayers are said and a chant begins, spiritual energies invoked to balance the intensity of the earthly experience.

Some people seem to just soak up the ambience and emerge glowing. Others may burst into tears, releasing pent-up fears and hostilities. A good ceremony releases disharmony on all levels; pockets of held-in negative energies are driven out by the heat and the ritual, allowing people to fill their bodies and minds with new pure energies. The heat itself may also be useful, for it raises the body's temperature, which kills some kinds of pathogenic organisms and induces certain immune system functioning, the same way a fever does.

As you emerge from the sweat lodge into the chilled night air, with a canopy of sparkling stars overhead, clouds of steam rise from your sweating body. Some people call it a night after one round. Others may throw a bucket of cold water over themselves or jump into a cold lake or stream and then repeat the process. In the Scandinavian saunas, which operate traditionally in a very similar fashion to Indian sweat lodges, people roll in the snow or beat each other with slender birch wands to stimulate circulation after each time inside the heat.

According to Brooke, sweats cultivate the power of "seeing," or becoming more aware of the present, knowing what's best for you, and becoming better able to anticipate the future. Images of the red-and-black paintings of the Pacific Northwest Coast Indians come to mind, which depict eyes throughout the entire bodies of people, animals, and trees.

Another nature healer with a foot in both modern and traditional worlds is Lewis Mehl of Tucson, Arizona. Lewis received instruction in traditional Cherokee healing methods growing up in Oklahoma and then went on to get an M.D. from Stanford and a Ph.D. in clinical psychology. Calling upon his experience in modern and ancient methods, Lewis frequently prescribes sweat-lodge ceremonies for patients with many different types of cancer, drug addictions, and even some people with AIDS. In one memorable case of a man who was HIV-positive, Mehl reports that a spirit of a thunderbird came to the sweat lodge and spoke with the ill man, instructing him to go outside in a pouring rain, strip down nude, and pray in a *heyoka,* or contrary, fashion—that is, to pray for everything he didn't want to have happen. The threat of AIDS moved him to do just this, and he stood naked in the rain and started to scream out that he wanted to die. As the words came out, he broke into deep sobs, and to his amazement his immune system soon became stronger. Mehl explains that this procedure gave voice to all those parts that were resisting being healthy, which released them from his unconscious mind, allowing him to face and defeat them rather than denying that they existed, which was a root cause of his illness.

Becoming a truly adept nature healer is not something one accomplishes overnight. The masters of nature healing slowly grow into their skill, almost always going through a process of personal healing of an illness that seems to descend upon them as a cosmic lesson that must be learned before embarking on a profession of healing. A look at three of the best of such healers sheds light on the vast potential of this little-understood aspect of human nature.

THREE MASTER NATURE HEALERS

HAWAIIAN KAHUNA MORRNAH SIMEONA

Morrnah Nalamaku Simeona is a Kahuna *Lapa'au* (master sha-man) who lives on Oahu in Hawaii. She is descended from generations of kahunas who served the kings and queens of Hawaii long before it became a state. They say that Morrnah showed the first signs of her calling when she was four. She talked to spirits she could see and then placed her hands on people and took away their headaches. In recognition of her lifelong service to the people of Hawaii and of the world (she has given workshops on traditional methods of healing and peace-making for the United Nations), Morrnah has been declared a "Living Treasure" by the state of Hawaii. After my first visit to see her in 1978, I began to understand why.

Morrnah and I met at her comfortable offices in the Founda-tion of I, which she has formed to carry on the ancient art of *Ho'oponopono,* a traditional Hawaiian approach to healing and conflict resolution. In Morrnah's view the source of all health and dis-ease in the world is related to rhythms—inside of us, between us and nature, and in the world around us. The clouds, the birds singing, the warm earth underfoot, the steady lapping of waves on the sandy shore—each of these forces of nature in the world around us has a special natural rhythmic frequency. The traditional Hawaiian way of speaking, "talking story," helps to communicate the feeling of this wisdom, for if you are in tune with nature, then your language also has a rhythm, and if you weave your words together correctly, a conversation casts a spell and conveys a blessing.

We discussed Hawaiian traditions about nature and sacred places for some time. As our conversation was coming to a close, Morrnah pointed to some very large fern plants growing outside her window in the courtyard. "Sometimes the spirits of things get inside people and disturb their harmonies," she said. "The spirit of a thing is more powerful in healing than its body in this world sometimes."

That night I had a vivid dream in which Morrnah appeared in a long flowing robe. She walked over to me, and from her eyes came beams of light, like flashlights shining right through me. I felt as though she were conducting an examination. Then she reached out her hand, and it went into me. She pulled out a thing that looked like a dead fern plant. Then she picked some fronds from some fresh, vital ferns growing nearby and placed them back into my body in the area where she had extracted the dead ones. In my dream I heard a lullaby. The next day, when I awoke, a muscle spasm associated with an old football injury, which had flared up from the long plane ride to Hawaii, had disappeared. Morrnah just chuckles about this, saying that we can heal with our *amakua,* or spirit double, as well as we can in this physical plane. Right actions, by themselves, represent a prayer for health and wholeness, she later reminded me. (See the Appendix for more information about Morrnah Simeona.)

RAONI OF THE AMAZON RAIN FOREST

In January 1986 the life of Brazilian naturalist Augusto Ruschi was ebbing away due a liver ailment. During a research trip through the rain forests he had touched a deadly poisonous Dendrobates toad. Modern medicine knew no cure. In desperation Brazilian president José Sarney sent out a call for Raoni, the noted medicine man of the Txucarramae tribe, which lives in the remote Xingu National Park. Raoni and another medicine man named Sapaim from the nearby Caimura tribe were flown to Brasilia, where the seventy-year-old scientist lay dying.

Raoni said that in a dream he had seen Ruschi struggling with a horde of poisonous toads. If he wasn't treated properly, Raoni said, Ruschi would become like a toad and die. Pictures of the naturalist's bloated face confirmed the shaman's diagnosis.

Raoni and Sapaim began their therapy by blowing smoke from ten-inch-long cigars on the patient, chanting, and praying. After a time it seemed that the medicine man appeared to reach into the scientist and extract what a *New York Times* reporter present described as a "green, strong-smelling pasty substance," which Raoni said was "toad poison." They gave Ruschi an herbal bath, and after three more days of doctoring him they declared him cured.

At a press conference not long after the healing, a glowing Ruschi proclaimed, "I feel as I have never felt before. White men can learn a lot from Indians." Ruschi went on to voice his support for saving the rain forests and their indigenous peoples, and concluded his statement with the conviction that "the hummingbirds will lead you to God."[13]

ROLLING THUNDER

In August 1982, just east of Seattle, Washington, not far from Snoqualmie Falls, I watched Rolling Thunder manifest an awesome display of spiritual healing for a client of mine who was diagnosed as having multiple sclerosis (MS). Because of my friendship with Rolling Thunder, and because the woman was my client, I was able to observe the healing process that took place between them over a two-month period.

Despite the many advances of modern medicine some illnesses remain a mystery. Multiple sclerosis is one of these. First described in modern medical literature by Jean-Martin Charcot in 1872, MS has no known cause or cure. It's essentially a set of associated symptoms, characterized as a progressively worsening degeneration of the central nervous system, that affects some 500,000 people in the United States. Typically it appears between the ages of twenty and forty as a numbness or partial paralysis of one or more of the limbs, transient blindness, and associated malfunctioning of the nervous system. From onset to death the duration is typically ten to twenty years, with progressive loss of bodily functioning. Death is usually by suffocation, although many people become despondent and commit suicide. Once in a great while MS will spontaneously disappear for no apparent reason.

The woman Rolling Thunder treated was middle-aged. Three and a half years earlier she had begun to notice some loss of strength in her legs. A physician diagnosed her as having MS and placed her on a schedule of conventional physical therapy. The weakness in her legs grew worse, slowly spreading to her arms and hands. After about a year and a half she was not getting any better, so she was referred to a special center for people with MS. She was shocked. "They all seemed as if they were just waiting around to die," she said, and walked out determined she would not follow that path. She left her doctor and began to explore alternative-treatment methods. She experienced some short-lived symptomatic relief from chiropractic and acupuncture, but her overall condition didn't improve.

For nearly a month I saw her twice a week, sometimes for two hours at a time, using all the techniques in imagery, Gestalt, and counseling I knew. Although she gained new insights into herself and her depression began to go away, the physical symptoms didn't improve. She also tried working with other therapists, who used massage and other somatic therapies, but she didn't experience any significant change in her symptoms.

"Healing is a matter of time, but it is also a matter of opportunity," Hippocrates once said. It turned out the woman was part Indian. I told her that Rolling Thunder would be coming to town in two months and asked if she was interested in consulting with him. She said she had read the book about him by Doug Boyd and that she certainly was interested.

I warned her that a medicine person works differently from a medical doctor. Rolling Thunder will only "doctor" a person if he receives guidance from the Great Spirit. She said she understood. I suggested she send him a gift of tobacco, along with a letter describing her condition and why she wanted to be healthy again. She sent off her request to Carlin, Nevada, where Rolling Thunder lives.

Three days later, approximately the amount of time it takes for a first-class parcel to travel from Seattle to Carlin, she had an extremely vivid dream. Standing at the foot of her bed were two figures. One was wearing a flowing black robe and looked like Darth Vader from the *Star Wars* movies. The other was a large pink caterpillar. She awoke frightened and charged with so much energy that she couldn't sleep the rest of the night.

The next afternoon she fell asleep on a couch and had another vivid dream. This time she was standing inside a supermarket with Rolling Thunder right beside her. He produced a magic carpet, which he spread before her, and invited her to get on it. She did, and they flew off together around the world. When they got back, Rolling Thunder gave her a hug and a kiss. She awoke and found that she could get up and move around the house for about an hour with more ease than she had known in a long time.

When Rolling Thunder arrived in town two months later, the lady with MS had become strong enough that she and a friend cooked for Rolling Thunder's party. When they met, she gave him a beautiful hand-carved pipe and some tobacco. From the outset Rolling Thunder made it clear that regardless of what she did, he could only help her as much as the Great Spirit would allow.

The first evening he said he would like to talk with the woman. The party was staying in a two-level chalet made from an old barn. Rolling Thunder's room was on the second floor. He remained in his room, requesting that the woman come to see him—and no one was to give her any help getting up the stairs. Slowly, painfully, she climbed the stairs on her hands and knees. The message was very clear from the beginning that if she was going to get better, she was going to have to work at it with great determination.

Their first meeting lasted nearly an hour, with Rolling Thunder asking her a series of questions that represented a very thorough case history, just as any physician would do. At the end of this time he puffed on his corncob pipe, made some suggestions about her diet, and said he'd have to consult with the spirits. Then some people with Rolling Thunder brought up a drum and sang several songs for her.

Several days later Rolling Thunder held his second session. Again the woman had to climb the stairs by herself. Accompanied by a chiropractor, Rolling Thunder performed a series of subtle physical manipulations of the woman's body. In the process of this examination, which was conducted on a massage table, the woman fell asleep. When this happened, Rolling Thunder asked us to leave the room. As we did, he settled down into a big easy chair next to the woman and closed his eyes.

Downstairs a group of people were talking and drinking coffee. While it was still early, people seemed to become drowsy, and the pace of activity slowed down as a soft cloud of energy filled the room. All but two of us fell asleep, as if we'd been drugged. It seemed as though Rolling Thunder's physical examination had also placed the woman in a trance, which he then entered. His mind field was strong enough that the "spell" of his trance filled the entire chalet, pulling most of those present into its ambience. Half an hour later Rolling Thunder quietly came down the stairs. There was a tear in his voice as he said, "She's had a rough time in life," and then he walked out the door into a grove of giant red cedars nearby, coughing.

Several days later, at the conclusion of his workshop, Rolling Thunder said that the Great Spirit had given him the approval to perform a healing ceremony later that day, and everyone who had attended the workshop was invited to stay. None of the sixty people present left.

"Medicine people don't do things for show," Rolling Thunder said to the crowd as an hour later he emerged from the chalet. Then he added, "But there's a right time and place for everything." On his head was a navy blue hat, or turban as he called it, with several eagle feathers hanging down from it at odd angles. Above his forehead was a silver seven-pointed-star pin with a large turquoise stone set in the middle. Circles painted in a white chalky substance were on his cheeks. He said they represented the Grandmother Moon and the Grandfather Sun. Painted on his forehead was a simple tree symbol with upturned branches. This, he said, was the Cherokee Tree of Life.

He was wearing a black vest decorated with an elaborate floral beadwork pattern characteristic of the eastern Indian tribes. Rolling Thunder was a sturdy six feet tall, with the muscular build of a football quarterback, and perhaps the most striking article of all was a full badger skin hanging from his waist. The skin had been fashioned into a medicine bag, and from the badger's open mouth protruded an eagle-feather wand.

Two of his helpers, Cloud Lightning and Alan, set up a large powwow drum in a nearby forest clearing. They asked us to form a circle, and soon we began to chant a welcoming song: "Hey hey, hey hey, unduwah." As our voices rose together, Rolling Thunder stepped into the circle and taught us a simple dance, the Cherokee Two-Step. As we circled around chanting, Rolling Thunder walked to the center of the circle and offered a prayer to the Great Spirit, the four directions, the earth mother, and the spiritual forces. He sent out a puff of smoke to each power as we now stood in the silence, broken only by the whisper of the wind through the branches of the giant aromatic cedars and the distant chortle of a raven.

As we continued to chant and dance, Rolling Thunder took off his badger-skin medicine bag and his boots. He looked skyward, his lips moving slightly in prayer. When he again looked at us, his face and eyes had a cold, piercing quality, like the gaze of an eagle. He began to dance in the circle, slowly at first, arms outstretched like wings, like an eagle floating in circles on a warm summer updraft. Gradually his pace quickened until it became frenzied and energetic far beyond one's expectations for a person of his sixty-seven years. At the height of this dance his eyes met mine for an instant, and to my amazement what I saw for just a flash was a being half-eagle and half-man. A moment later he suddenly stopped and let out an ear-splitting *whoop!* As if the dance had been choreographed, instantly everyone stopped dancing and chanting. Changing his composure, Rolling Thunder jokingly said, "You didn't tell me you were all Indians." Laughter rippled around the circle. Nearly forty-five minutes had gone by since we began, I noted, checking my watch. Rolling Thunder then asked us to move to a second circle around a fire that had been built nearby.

The drummers picked up their beat again at the second circle as another helper, Mike Thor, moved around the circle with a smudge of sweetgrass and sage, directing the smoke with an eagle feather to each person, first to our hearts, then over the top of our heads, purifying body, mind, and spirit. Again we began to chant.

Rolling Thunder emerged from the chalet carrying a wool blanket and an old suitcase. He spread the blanket in the center of the circle, opened the suitcase, and took out an eagle-feather wand and a buffalo-tail whisk, as well as a strange collection of objects, including stones and crystals, which he arranged into a simple altar on the blanket. Shamans in South America call this their *mesa,* which means table. Its purpose is to create a "microcosm of the macrocosm," a design pattern with objects that establish a series of harmonic links to the spirit world, pulling in energies to create a powerful spiritual ambience and a guiding beacon for right action. In the intensity of a ceremony this mesa "rises," according to shamans, if the spirit is strong enough. To see it rise, you have to learn to look at it "kinda out of the corner of your eye," Rolling Thunder says.

Then a jug of water was brought to him. The water had been obtained during an earlier ceremony at a sacred spring.

At this point the woman was led out of the chalet. She was wrapped in a blanket, wearing only her underpants and an eagle feather in her hair. She moved very slowly, with the aid of a cane and the help of two women, who helped her to lie down on a blanket and covered her.

Rolling Thunder picked up his buffalo-tail whisk and walked around the woman, brushing the ground around her and her body, clearing away negative energies. Then he put down the buffalo-tail whisk and picked up the eagle-feather wand. Again he circled her, this time making graceful brushing strokes in the air above her. Then he stood back and raised the wand into the air in each of the four directions, and then directed the wand toward her body, calling in the powers of directions for support.

Satisfied with the purification, he put down the wand and stood in silent prayer, looking upward. Then he raised his right hand up into the air, gesturing to the world above. He brought his left hand to his mouth and spit into it. Then he let out an ear-piercing *whoop* and slapped his hands together. He stood there for a moment staring at his hands. Then he knelt down and slid his hands under the blanket and placed them on the woman's body for a minute or two.

Then he repeated the spitting, clapping, and whooping process. This time, as he held his hands up before his face, I seemed to see a purple glow around his hands and head, like the kind of radiant glow you see around holy people in spiritual paintings. Again he laid his hands on her body for two to three minutes as we all sang to a heartbeat drum rhythm.

Rolling Thunder now stood again and said silent prayers, and this time, when he looked at us, his eyes glared with an animal-like quality. He got down on all fours beside the woman and began to whine, growl, and sniff. He was now a badger-human in search of his prey, the way a real-life badger would hunt a mouse. He circled her, slowly, searching for a scent. Then his actions became more animated, and his whining grew louder. Honing in on her lower back, he now began to growl and picked up her blanket and thrust his head underneath. The sounds that then came forth sounded like a badger in a fever pitch of excitement. He placed his mouth on her back and began to suck. In a few moments he pulled back and motioned for someone to bring him a bowl. He coughed up something that looked like green pus. Then he repeated the sucking and vomiting several times until he could only cough up clear liquid.

As he was finishing the sucking, a giant black-and-orange wood wasp of the ichneumonid variety suddenly flew into the circle, seemingly headed straight for Rolling Thunder. This species has a body three to four inches long and a long trailing ovipositor of about the same length. The eight-inch wasp made two angry passes around Rolling Thunder and the woman. Rolling Thunder glared at it, and it suddenly flew off into the woods, as people in its line of flight scattered in terror.

Now clearly tired, Rolling Thunder got to his feet and again brushed the area around the woman with his buffalo-tail whisk. He motioned for the two women helpers to come and help the woman get up. They helped her into a chair. Her face was radiant as she smiled with a warmth and strength I'd never seen before. The drumming stopped, and silence hung in the air. All eyes were on her as she exclaimed, "I am alive!" and rose to her feet. Rolling Thunder handed her her cane, and the women with her started to help her go back to the chalet. After a few steps she tossed away the cane. Her helpers let go of her, and she proceeded to walk all the way back unaided as we all cheered wildly. All around the circle people were hugging each other and crying.

"Today this woman's been healed," Rolling Thunder said with authority. "I don't mean cured, but healed. If she leads a good life, walking the good red road, eats the right things, and takes care of herself, she'll live a long time. She'll need to be doctored again, by me or someone else like me, and if she does, she'll walk too. This is the Great Spirit's way. I didn't heal her, the Great Spirit did. I was just the Great Spirit's agent, that's all. Ho!"

As I was standing and talking to others who'd seen the ceremony, six people independently came up to me and asked me if I'd seen the purple glow around Rolling Thunder's head and hands.

Later the woman told me that during the ceremony she had kept her thoughts positive, as Rolling Thunder had instructed. While lying on the ground, she had a vision of herself walking along a path and then starting to dance. Her first step on this new path was to walk around unaided for an hour or so, the first time she'd been able to walk that way in years.

Several hours later she needed the cane again, but it was obvious she had much more strength. A week later she said she was having "ups and downs," but was feeling much better. Three years later she reported to me that she was not totally free of the cane but was strong enough to hold down a part-time job. For recreation she swam three times a week and went horseback riding twice weekly. She said that the "Indian part" of her was taking over, and as it did, she felt more and more "love for nature, animals, rocks, and the Great Spirit." Then I lost track of her.

In Rolling Thunder's model all real healing begins on the spiritual plane, then works its way down into the mental plane and finally into the physical plane. Rolling Thunder first invoked the spirit of the eagle for guidance. Then as he worked on the physical plane he took on the grounding power of the buffalo for protection before he finally went to battle as a badger. During that afternoon he was a living totem pole of spirits, aided by allies such as the spring water, the crystals on his mesa, the giant cedar trees, and the nearby spirit of Snoqualmie Falls. Bringing together his allies through ceremonies, Rolling Thunder became what Carl Jung termed a "mana person," someone of awesome personal power, a living archetype.

Rolling Thunder later told me that "black magic" had been involved in her illness, meaning that an intrusive force from someone else's mind had entered her mind-body system, creating disharmony and illness. Knowing her life story, I would say this was true, for several people had done horrible things to her on a psychic and physical level. The appearance of the giant wood wasp at that time in the ceremony represented a manifestation of the evil that had been used against her, he said. Animals can be messengers of light or dark forces.

Each of us has certain healing abilities, but to be able to perform a ceremony like this requires a special calling, Rolling Thunder asserts. "You can't copy another person's medicine," Rolling Thunder told me later. "You get your medicine powers as gifts, one by one, slowly. They can be taken away, too, if you abuse them."

BEAUTY AND HEALTH

When Knud Rasmussen traveled among the Eskimos in the early 1900s, he met a shaman named Otaq, who told him, "I do not want to die, because it is good to live"[14]—such a different attitude than living because of the fear of death.

Studying the oldest people on earth, Dr. Alexander Leaf, of Harvard University Medical School, found several common elements in their lives regardless of whether they lived in the mountains, at the equator, or beside the Arctic Ocean: plenty of physical exercise, not necessarily as a regimen, but more often as part of the regular daily lifestyle; a simple diet, generally with some meat; loving support and respect from the community where they live; and usually a healthy sex life.[15]

Another ingredient of health and longevity that needs to be added is the ability to see and appreciate beauty in the world around you. Richard Nelson reports that the Koyukon Indians of Alaska "see their environment not only as a source of life and spiritual power, but also a world of beauty." Nelson relates,

> A man spent several minutes describing a particular midwinter sunset, its color glowing on the frozen river and the snow-covered mountainside, snow on the trees reflecting

amber, and long shadows cast by timber on the slopes. He said his wife had called him out so he could see it, and he stood a long time watching. Both he and his wife are old, and he says that the oldest people during his childhood had this same admiration for beauty.[16]

"There is good reason to believe that the patient's state of mind can affect the course of all pathological processes that involve immunological reactions," René Dubos said. The power of natural beauty to inspire us to be healthy and happy cannot be overstated. According to physician Bernie Siegel in his best-selling book *Love, Medicine and Miracles,* "The ambiance of the clinical environment influences the attitude of both doctor and patient. I fear that we lost one of our most important sources of strength—a connection to God and nature—when hospital planning took the windows out.... A view of the outside world reminds us of our link to nature."[17]

It comes as no great surprise, then, that when Kenneth Pelletier examined the lives of people who recovered from serious illness despite great odds, they all shared a deep sense of the importance of the spiritual as well as the material aspects of life.[18] Realizing the power of nature to move us to health and happiness, the truth of the Navajo chanter's words, "In beauty may you walk, my grandchild, Thus will it be beautiful," becomes obvious.

FINDING YOUR OWN NATURE HEALER

The Greek healer Asklepios supposedly entered Athens in 420 B.C. accompanied by his ally, the snake, which curled around his staff, forming the symbol for modern medicine, the caduceus. The snake is seen as a symbol of sexuality as well as earth-force energy and the kundalini spiritual energy that Hindu mystics say lies at the base of the spine waiting to ascend to bring about enlightenment. As the staff implies, the cultivation of the basic primal life force and its elevation upward to unite with the conscious mind is the way healing wisdom is cultivated.

A temple to honor Asklepios was then erected on the southern slope of the Acropolis, not far from some springs that are still thought to have healing powers today. Inspired by Asklepios, the following journey is one you can take to gain insights into your own natural healer, as well as your needs.

Set yourself up in a comfortable place where you can relax for fifteen to twenty minutes, as you go on the following journey. (If you want a tape of this journey with special music, see the back of the book for details.)

This is a journey in search of a nature healer who is especially suited for you. Begin by seeing yourself walking down a path through a field, at the end of which is a hill, surrounded by a forest. The path continues into the forest and around the hill. Notice how you negotiate the hill. Do you go to the left or right, or even climb over the top? When you get to the other side of the hill, you will find a building that is the temple of your nature healer. Note its shape and architecture.

When you come to the temple, before entering make an offering of some food beside the trail, honoring the spirits of nature who are working with you. You may also want to say a prayer. When you enter the temple, you will find your guide to nature healing. Introduce yourself and tell the guide why you are there.

Now the guide will take you down into a sacred mine. Together you go down, down into the earth, until you reach a place where you come to a sacred gem or mineral. Examine the healing stone. You may want to ask the guide how to use it.

After you have become familiar with the healing stone, bring it back up to the surface with you. Ask your guide about the stone and how it can help you. Say good-bye to your guide, and then exit from the temple. Walk back on the path until you come back into the field again. Then let go of the scene and return to your experience of the room and your body. You can

return to the healing temple again anytime you like, to ask
your guide other questions about health and healing.

Comments: The gemstone symbolizes the anchoring powers
of the mineral kingdom. The more sensitive you become, the
more you must ground yourself to keep your center as you
process more information. Gems also act as transformers of
energy, giving you the channel or frequency you need. A bright-
red ruby has different qualities of powers than a deep-blue
sapphire or a purple amethyst, for example.

You can return to your nature healer and the temple at any
time for additional consultations. Many people find that this
exercise helps to ground them and make them more stable and
consistent. As always, if you have any symptoms of a physical
illness, you should consult a medical doctor of your choice.

One day I did this exercise for a young boy who was battling
leukemia. His conventional treatments weren't working that
well, so we talked about how his chemotherapy and his natural
immune system were working against the cancerous cells in his
blood. I guided him into the natural-healing temple, and after a
few minutes I asked him what he'd found there to help him. I
had expected he'd say a he found a bear or a lion. Instead he said
with a rush of energy, "A big green tank!" We laid out pillows
on the floor to symbolize his diseased cells. Then he became the
big green tank and jumped up and down on them with a frenzy
until he became exhausted. His mother went out and bought him
a green toy tank, which sat beside his bed. His recovery shortly
took a quantum leap forward, and the last I heard, his leukemia
had gone into remission.

Chapter Seven

THE SPIRIT OF PLACE

*The earth is the origin of all things,
the root and the garden of all life; the place
where all things, the beautiful, the ugly,
the good and the bad, the foolish and
the clever come into being.*

—JOSEPH NEEDHAM
Science and Civilization in China

Over a memorable dinner with Joseph Campbell a few years ago, I asked the eminent mythologist which places around the world were most special to him. With little hesitation he replied that Delphi, the caves at Lascaux in France, and Palenque in Mexico were his most favorite places. I asked Campbell why these places were so special to him. He took a sip of wine, looked out the window for a long moment, and then turned and said to me, "Because I, Joe Campbell, felt more powerful there, and I damn well don't know why!"

After working among the Navajo of the American Southwest for many years, Francis Newcomb and Gladys Reichard observed,

Locality is of the utmost importance among the Navajo. Names of people, of animals, of dangers, names of arrows, of lightnings and plants, have power when known and used properly; even so names of places are charms. Just as the modern writer or dramatist gives his work setting, so also

does the Navajo myth. Whenever a protagonist meets someone who is powerful the first question he must answer is
"where do you come from?"[1]

Entering Colorado from southwestern Utah on Utah State
Highway 262—a dirt and gravel upgraded wagon road that leads
you through herds of sheep, dry washes lined with groves of
cottonwoods, and past beehive-shaped Navajo hogans—two
promontories rise to greet you. To the south lies Sleeping Ute
Mountain, a giant resting warrior who influences local weather,
according to the Ute Mountain tribe. To the east looms the dark-
green, flat-topped plateau of Mesa Verde, abruptly rising up
some two thousand feet. Most people say they visit Mesa Verde
to see the spectacular ancient cliff dwellings. But there is something else there, too—the power of place.

The literature of Mesa Verde National Park describes the
Anasazi Indians, who populated Mesa Verde for seven hundred
years until they vanished in the late 1200s. On the flyer is a
striking photo of the Cliff Palace pueblo tucked under a canyon
rim. Even more interesting is the park's slogan at the bottom of
the page, Where the Spirits Rise.

I ask the ranger about the "spirits," and he points me to the
bar at the Far View Lodge—a good place to think about spirits,
but not quite what I had in mind. Consulting my *Funk and
Wagnall's Standard Dictionary,* I find twenty-odd definitions
ranging from spirituality to discarnate entities, liquor, the excitement of a group of people, and the way a place feels. Aside from
the use of "spirit" to describe alcohol, most of the other nineteen
definitions concern a magical vital quality that cannot be
smelled, seen, tasted, or heard but can be sensed and has an
influence on human behavior. The preferred definition is, "The
principle of life and energy in man and animals, at one time
regarded as being composed of an extremely refined substance,
such as breath or warm air, separable from the body, mysterious
in nature, and ascribable to a definite origin."

Scholars can talk forever about what is spirit, but the unique experience of place is something you must feel in your bones. The place where we were born and raised is a touchstone of renewal to every person. Other places, too, have a special call to our senses. The ancient Greeks sited their temple to honor Gaia, the earth goddess, at Delphi. Their selection of this site was not by chance. Sages said that at Delphi a mysterious life force called the plenum bubbles up out of the ground. The abundance of the plenum at Delphi favors prophecy, they asserted, so temples to honor Greek gods and goddesses, including Gaia, were constructed among Delphi's craggy rocks and rugged hills, honoring the spirit of place.

In 1984 the First World Congress on Cultural Parks was held at Mesa Verde National Park, assembling people from fifty countries all around the world to discuss heritage preservation. One afternoon a group of people representing traditional cultures gathered around a table. Everyone was happy to be there, but universally they felt modern people didn't seem to understand why traditional cultures feel places have special spirit and power.

Brian Hounseal, a landscape architect working with the Huna Indians of Central American, stood up and said that the ancient Greeks had a concept they called the genius loci, or the "spirit of place," which was the cornerstone of their approach to land planning. Hounseal said if we really understood the spirit of place, maybe modern society could understand ancient earth wisdom better. Everyone around the table nodded agreement. As one of those seated around that table, in that moment I recalled a dream I had had several years earlier in which Mad Bear Anderson had appeared and suggested that someday I should organize a conference about special places on the earth. Putting this dream together with that magic moment at Mesa Verde, the "Spirit of Place" symposium series was conceived.

When I returned home, I went to research what had been written about the subject. I found two books in the massive

University of California library system that contained the "spirit of place" concept, both diaries by British authors—Alice Meynard in 1899 and D. H. Lawrence in 1923, reflecting their impressions of how different places influenced them. A master with words, Lawrence wrote, "Different places on the face of the earth have different vital effluence, different vibration, different chemical exhalation, different polarity with different stars: call it what you like but the spirit of place is a great reality."[2]

You can't fully appreciate the spirit of a place by intellectualizing it, you have to let it creep into your body and allow it to cast a spell on your soul.

The "Spirit of Place" program began in 1987 with a widely circulated Call for Papers, publicized in many places, including the *Chronicle of Higher Education* (but not *Science* magazine), requesting proposals for papers that would address traditional cultural wisdom about place and its relevance to modern society. Over 150 proposals were submitted, and 70 papers were finally accepted. Similar formats were used for the 1989 program at Grace Cathedral in San Francisco and the 1990 symposium, which returned to Mesa Verde National Park.

Some 185 speakers participated in these three "Spirit of Place" symposiums—architects, attorneys, Indians, Eskimos, Africans, space scientists, landscape architects, psychologists, geomancers, priests, activists, physicists, engineers, scholars, and a representative of a commune. While the speakers were extremely diverse in background and lifestyle, they all agreed on the importance of a subject that wasn't even supposed to exist. At the risk of oversimplifying, the following are my own interpretations of their conclusions:

1. For indigenous cultures all around the world, the belief in the existence of certain places having a special sacred value or power is seemingly universal and frequently a cornerstone of meaning and cultural behaviors. Little is known about why people are so attracted to special places, but their spell still

works on us, too. One of the most common of all world-tourism motives is the desire to visit special, even sacred, places.

2. Traditional cultures have many different types of sacred places, which seem to serve as special amplifiers of certain facets of consciousness—fertility, initiation, seeking dreams, burial, rituals, healing, and so on—just as we have books that deal with different subjects. The collective power of these many different kinds of places serves to energize the human mind into a state of unitive, intuitive consciousness, in which the boundaries between the spiritual and material planes of life are less clear—in the Salish tribe's tongue, *skalalitude.*

3. In the United States and other modern countries, special places are protected for society as a whole as sacred places only if they are the sites of man-made structures, such as churches and shrines or cemeteries. Otherwise they are archeological treasures, relics from the past and to other people.

4. Most countries recognize that some places may have sacred value to traditional cultures, but seldom are these places legally recognized as being sacred to modern society, even though all of us are descended from cultures that revere certain special sacred places in nature.

5. One of the principal characteristics of sacred places, according to traditional cultures, is that they contain an extra "energy." A growing body of modern scientific research documents the existence of subtle environmental fields (electromagnetic fields, air ions, and so on) that can influence plants, animals, and people, and some data document the fact that unusual environmental fields may be found at certain sacred places. Other places also have unique soil and water chemistry, but it's uncertain if there are any consistent scientific measurements that can determine what is a sacred place.

6. The world's most famous architecture has been designed with the aid of geomancy, the spiritual parent of modern environmental design. There are many cases where the ancient art and

science of geomancy has been applied to modern home and work settings with positive results. Modern science has not yet been able to explain why many of these geomantic cures seem to work, but that shouldn't stop people from using them.

7. Most people experience places as having different feelings or personalities, and some places seem to be capable of deeply inspiring people to make pilgrimages to them, where they may have experiences of a mystical or transpersonal nature. Traditional cultures believe that "sacred sites are for the protection of all people" (quoted from a message from the Northern Cheyenne elders).

8. Some people seem to become "voices" for certain places, and frequently they do not consciously understand why. When they do become an advocate for a place, they often feel deeply moved to express their feelings in art and action. Psychologist Robert Sommer said at the conference, "Like others here, I am a spokesman for a place, and I cannot say how or why I was chosen for this role."

9. Perception of the subtle qualities of place is of the utmost importance to excellence in landscape planning, but in modern times this is not well understood. For many gifted landscape architects, such as Lawrence Halprin, the spirit of place is captured in sketches and impressions more easily than in words, in part because we don't have a good vocabulary to express our sense of place. Eskimos have numerous words for ice and snow, and Polynesians have many different words and phrases for waves and water. We value land highly, but we explain this value monetarily. We must find a better way to articulate the unique qualities of place and translate them into design, for this is critical to design excellence. As former California state architect Sim Van der Ryn stated, "I want to be a part of a culture where the spirit of place is a part of everyone's language, experience, and practice."

10. Modern society generally sees nature as something "out there" in the woods or in the deepest African jungles. Re-

gardless of where we are, whether in the heart of Manhattan or in Detroit, in the Brooks Range of Alaska or the grassy plains of South Dakota, the spirit of that place influences us. We may separate ourselves from nature in our language, but not in reality.

In his review of the "Spirit of Place" program for *Earth Island Journal,* Jonathon Bates described the program thus: "In September 1988, in the heat of California's Indian Summer, amidst the deep shade of the tree-lined campus of the University of California at Davis, a new environmental discipline was born."

The first part of this book has presented a system for increasing personal awareness and harmony with nature and anchoring our intuitional roots there. To make living in harmony with nature a reality, you need to begin with where your feet touch the ground and to take this awareness and translate it into a lifestyle that makes your life work best in a series of ever-growing circles of reality—home, neighborhood, work, community, state, nation, world.

SUGGESTION: What are your favorite places? If you could go anyplace in the world, what three places would you like to visit? Write them down and then add a couple of sentences on why you would like to visit them. In a similar fashion, is there a place in nature within one mile of your house that you particularly like? It can be even a single tree. Can you explain why this place feels special to you? Visit it.

UNDERSTANDING PLACE

Studies show that most Americans spend 75 percent of their lives indoors. Frank Lloyd Wright used to claim he could build a house that would guarantee a divorce in six months. Recent research on colors, textures, lighting, sounds, and electromagnetic fields and their influence on our moods, mind, health, and

behavior supports Wright's claim and makes one wonder why
we put up with what Wright called cash-and-carry architecture.

No one understands the negative aspects of modern artificial
environments better than Debra Dadd. At twenty-four Dadd was
a talented pianist for the San Francisco Opera. Just as her career
was beginning to take off, she fell victim to a strange set of
worsening, debilitating symptoms including insomnia, muscle
aches, depression, binge eating, and partial paralysis of her hands.
Fortunately her father recognized her problem as chemical sensitivity, a diagnosis confirmed by a physician. Her symptoms were
allergic reactions, attributable to trace substances, especially pe-
trochemicals such as the formaldehyde in permanent-press bed
sheets and polyester clothes; chlorine in the water she showered
with; and other substances in cleaning compounds, perfumes,
and synthetic fabrics. Survival, for Dadd, suddenly became determining the sources of her dis-ease in the world around her and
how to replace them with nourishing items.

Discovering that little information existed in a readily accessible form about chemically sensitive people, Dadd began her own
research program. As she grew better and better from removing
noxious substances in her environment, her sensitivity now enabled her to perceive the subtle pulses of nature. Soon she found
herself swept into transcendent reveries about life and nature
that have in turn fueled her commitment to rid the environment
of toxic substances. As a result she has become an expert in
toxic-free living and the author of popular books, including
Nontoxic and Natural and *The Nontoxic Home.*

According to the research of Marsha Adams of Woodside,
California, many people are also very sensitive to geophysical
factors, such as earthquakes. In addition to an aching big toe,
nausea, fatigue, irritability, and joint pains can show up in people
just before an earthquake. Since 1979 more than six hundred
people have contacted Adams's Time Research Institute to report symptoms that they associated with geophysical activity.
Working with these data and a select group of twenty sensitives,

Adams claims to have predicted the locations of earthquakes in the San Francisco Bay Area with an 85 percent to 90 percent accuracy and to have found some people who seem to sense quakes thousands of miles away.

One theory to account for this degree of sensitivity to the earth's field is that all humans have a small concentration of iron in the ethmoid bone, located at the base of the nose, right between the eyes. It's suspected that this is a rudimentary compass to help orient us to the earth's environmental fields. More than two dozen other animals have been found to possess a similar navigational system, suggesting that the earth's electromagnetic fields provide an orientation system that draws the web of life together with invisible threads as one potent element in the sense of place.

Over the last fifteen years my wife, a designer, and I have developed a system to help people gain greater awareness of the spaces they occupy so that they can make them more healthful and nourishing. This system is presented as a sequential process, starting from your physical body sense and moving outward into more and more subtle realities that collectively make up the environment around you.

DEVELOPING ENVIRONMENTAL SENSITIVITY

1. Listen to your own inner voice of environmental awareness.
Put on clothes made only from natural fabrics and go outside and find a place where you can sit comfortably on the ground and not be distracted. Take your shoes off and sit on the ground in a comfortable position. Close your eyes and take in a deep breath. Hold it for a few seconds and then let it out, making a sound if you like, to let go of any tension you may be carrying around. Do this two or three times. Now become aware of your body and mind. If you still find yourself tense, try performing the Sunshine Buddha exercise.

Keep your eyes closed and become aware of physical sensations such as how your body feels making contact with the earth. How does the sun, the wind, the temperature, and so on, feel on your body? Slowly open your eyes and look at the world around you in terms of textures and colors. Don't try to look at discrete images, just let them become a collage of sensations. Focus on the sensual experience of your body and of being alive.

If there is concrete or asphalt nearby, get up and walk over to the paved surface and stand there. Evaluate how your body feels. If you pay attention to your inner sensations, you'll probably find that your own inner energy field rises a little when it leaves direct contact with bare ground, making you a little less grounded. There's a lot of wisdom in the metaphor "down to earth."

If possible, go to a building and slowly go upward, floor by floor, continuing to be aware of your body. Some people will find that it becomes harder and harder to focus and concentrate as they get farther from the ground in man-made structures. If you feel uneasy in the mountains as well as in a high-rise building, that suggests fear of heights, but if you feel comfortable sitting on a mountain ledge looking at a river flowing by several hundred feet down and uneasy looking out the window of a high-rise the same height, you are probably field sensitive rather than afraid of heights. This is because some man-made structures disrupt the normal positive electrical charge of the earth, which we connect with through our feet. Feeling ungrounded in a high-rise building may be due to the loss of an electrical ground in your feet.

Each place you visit will cause a slightly different feeling in your body, which in turn brings out particular emotional feelings and thoughts. Is it coincidence that honeymooners go to Niagara Falls or spiritual pilgrims go to Jerusalem? At special places, such as Stonehenge, Mount Fuji, Machu Picchu, the Black Hills of South Dakota, and Denali, the natural fields are stronger, and research shows that when people walk into a strong environmental field, they bioentrain; that is, they harmonize with the external fields until inner biological rhythms and fields become identical with external ones.

2 *Refine your awareness of environmental conditions with a validity check.*

Wearing all-natural-fiber clothing, enlist the aid of a partner. Now raise one arm directly out in front of you until it is parallel to the ground. Tighten the muscles in your arm and have your partner push downward on your outstretched arm as you resist. Now take a tight-weave polyester-fabric shirt and just drape it over your shoulders. Again, put your arm out in front of you, tighten it, and have your partner push downward. Approximately 90 percent of the people I have tested with this procedure will find that their muscle strength is significantly weakened when the polyester shirt is on their body. This is due to electrical-field disruption, and the muscle weakness is symptomatic of a whole set of resulting symptoms produced by contact with substances that disrupt your personal fields. Take away the shirt, take a few deep breaths, and have your partner test you again—your muscle strength will be restored.

This test can be used for a wide variety of situations, for it is a very quick indication of the operating status of the body-mind system. For example, test yourself as a baseline and then put some white sugar in your other hand. Test your muscle strength again. Most people will be weakened by the sugar just contacting their bodies. For many people a weakening experience will occur if they place sugar within a foot of their body, close enough to be within their electromagnetic field.

When you feel you have the muscle test down, check out your strength both barefoot on your carpet and sitting on your furniture. Make a special point to test your muscle strength when you are sitting or lying on your bed. Humans spend about one third of their lives in bed, and many people wake up in the morning feeling exhausted due to what they've been sleeping on as much as what they've done the day before or how much sleep they've been getting. I've seen a number of women who have developed menstrual problems from sleeping on polyurethane-foam mattresses. In every case their sensitivity to the toxic effects of the mattress was indicated by muscle weakness. Other people have found that their carpet is the cause of tension headaches or that bed sheets can affect their health. You may even find that certain places in your house or place of work will cause your muscle strength to decrease. Be willing to consider that things such as electrical outlets, high-voltage power lines nearby, or structural features in the wall may be the cause. If you suspect that electro-magnetic-field pollution is the cause of your muscle weakness, you can buy small magnetic-field detectors for around two hundred dollars or less. Geiger counters in a similar price range are also available for checking out radiation, and radon-gas test kits are now on the market for twenty dollars or less. (See Appendix for details.)

When choosing colors or fabrics for your spaces, try using the muscle-testing system. Many people find that just looking at some colors will either strengthen or weaken their muscles. Remember, *you* have to live in the spaces you own or work in, not the designer.

3. Let your creative impressions flow.

Your house or office is a reflection of who you are. If the design somehow doesn't reflect your personality and tastes, you will be setting up intrapersonal and interpersonal conflicts due to the design's denial of yourself. Choose a room or a space in a room you would like to evaluate. Now take a sheet of paper and write, "I am this room, I am . . ." Now write a string of words and phrases that give a subjective impression of how this room feels to you, for example, "cool," "sloppy," "frenzied," "efficient." Reflect on this description of your space. Now start another sentence with "I would like this room to feel like . . ." and give a goal. Compare the two statements. We wholeheartedly endorse

Christopher Alexander in his classic book on interior design, *Pattern Language,* when he says, "Do not be tricked into believing that modern decor must be slick or psychedelic or 'modern art' or 'natural' or 'plants' or anything else that current tastemakers claim. It is most beautiful when it comes straight from your life—the things that tell your story."[3]

4. Use environmental harmonies to enliven your spaces.
Refer back to earlier exercises in which you found special plants and animals and ancestral links to nature. Can you include photos, paintings, or sculptures of them in your rooms? Make a list of your personal symbols of power from nature to use as a basis for weaving them into a design to make your house come into a harmony with nature that is most empowering for you. Shortly we'll discuss the *feng shui* system of geomancy, which will suggest ways of maximizing the value to your health of the placement of these artifacts.

Recall the special places you listed a moment ago. Are there ways of including them in your home by means of art objects? This will help to bring their presence more strongly into your daily life, in the same way that pictures of the family on the wall remind you of them. You can also extend this to your yard, perhaps, by planting shrubs or plants that remind you of these places.

5. Include your earth heritage in your home or yard.
The term "your family tree" is more than just an expression; it's one way of expressing your unique kinship with nature. Researching your genealogy, see if you can find examples of how special plants were used by your ancestors, the way the Gunn Clan of northern Scotland uses the juniper bush in many of their symbols and customs.

Each person is the product of a chain that reaches back to the earliest people, which is an important source of personal identity. Inside a home you could include ancestral plants and animals in art. In the surrounding yard, why not grow your family tree or plants associated with your ancestry?

One of the most cogent statements that has come out of the "Spirit of Place" symposium program was made by Vine Deloria, Jr., when he said, "A building should tell you everything about the society that you live in; its history, its possibilities, and its future." How does your home or office stack up against this standard? Does it create continuity with your past and future?

You may want to explore special designs of gardens for growing herbs or flowers also. Some people use stars, circles, or triangles to make their herb garden more harmonic or give it spiritual qualities. In many European traditions there is a belief that you should always leave a little part of your yard or garden wild, for "the little people."

DEVELOPING AND REFINING YOUR
PSYCHIC SENSE OF PLACE

On December 22, 1987, the National Research Council held a press conference to release a report of a three-year study commissioned by the National Academy of Sciences entitled "Enhancing Human Performance." One of the conclusions of the report was that "the committee finds no scientific justification from research conducted over 130 years for the existence of parapsychological phenomena."

You yourself may not have had any experiences such as clairvoyance, telepathy, or psychokinesis. If you haven't, please realize these experiences are considered normal, not paranormal, by far more people around the earth than those who see them as paranormal. To be sure, there are some definite fakes and sensationalists who profess to be psychics, but a blanket denial of the paranormal casts a vote against all the traditional cultures of the world and the wisdom they possess, as well as your own potential to better understand the significance of place.

The late Tuscarora Indian medicine man Mad Bear Anderson

was an expert on earth energies and a jolly, rotund man with an enormous personal energy field. Once he was approached by the New York State Highway Department and asked his opinion about a stretch of highway with an unusually high number of accidents. The design of this section of road had no physical features that could explain the number of accidents that took place there. Mad Bear went out and studied the area. His conclusion was that thousands of years ago a group of primitive hunters drove a herd of mastodons over a cliff at this site and killed them without performing the proper ceremonies to honor the spirits of the animals. The chaos of this event and the angered spirits of the animals still lurked in this valley, Mad Bear asserted, influencing people's judgment and concentration. He further told the astounded highway officials that if they wanted more proof, they could go to the American Museum of Natural History in New York and they'd find a skeleton of one of the animals there. That skeleton can actually be found there today.

Mad Bear then performed a ceremony to cleanse the area. Almost immediately the number of accidents in the area dropped dramatically.

A common parapsychological theatrical feat is to give a sensitive an object and then ask him or her to tell things about the owner or history of the object. This method of seeing is called psychometry, a word coined by Joseph Buchanan in 1842 to describe the process of reading the "soul" of a thing. Inspired by Mad Bear, I wondered if sensitives could shed light on the spirit of a place by just touching some soil.

The research procedure I developed calls for collecting small samples of soil with a clean trowel and putting each in a new container. The soil is not touched by the researcher's hands in order to ensure that his or her impressions are not encoded in it through contact. Soil samples are collected from a variety of places and tagged with randomly ordered labels. The samples are then delivered to a sensitive by a third party to avoid any face-to-face cues from the experimenter. The sensitives are asked to report their impressions of the places where the soils come from. I have performed this procedure with three different psychics, and in each case the results couldn't be explained by chance.

The first time I collected the soil samples at five sites on an automobile trip between Detroit and Seattle. The soil samples were then delivered to Dr. Mary Martin-Bacon, a noted sensitive in Seattle.

Her procedure for reading the soil was to assemble a group of ten of her best students and perform the readings as a group, each person reporting what they experienced when Dr. Bacon held some of the soil in her hand. The readings were recorded on a tape recorder. I never saw her or her students, nor did I even know when they assembled to do their reading. None of the samples had any special geological objects in them, such as unusual rocks or shells, that might give away their identity.

The first sample was taken from beneath a grove of mature Austrian black pine trees fifty to sixty years old, located right beside our family mineral well, the Wonder Well, on Grosse Ile, Michigan. Nearby there is a concrete-block building, as well as the bubbling well, which has had peak flows of two million gallons per day.

When this soil sample was assessed by the group, the following were some of their impressions:

"I feel there are six trees in the background and there's a pool." (Direct target hit!)

"I see a tower. It could be made of stone or rocks, or maybe clay. It seems like it is thirty feet high and about six feet in diameter." (The water comes out of the ground from just such a tower of stones, although it's not that tall anymore.)

A second soil sample was taken from a roadside park in the tiny town of Bassano, Alberta, which is on the eastern slope of the Canadian Rockies. We had stopped the car to stretch, and when we got back in the car, it wouldn't start. I climbed under the car and poked around. When I touched the solenoid with a screwdriver, a spark suddenly jumped and the car started. Apparently the car had collected too much static electricity and the car's ground was faulty. My touching the solenoid grounded out the car. In celebration of the moment I took a sample from the gravel beside the road. Some of the reports on this sample include:

"This is a totally different place from the first sample, it feels lonely, far from civilization, a far-from-life feeling. I also see an enormous ring or circle. It could be the edge of a crater or an adobe wall, but I'm inclined to think it's a rocky crater." (Bassano is a small town in the windswept high prairie. The gravel was no doubt taken from a quarry.)

"I don't get anything from the dirt, but whoever dug it up either got stung on the right hand or got stuck with something on the right hand when they were digging it or putting it into the bag." (The spark from the solenoid!)

The third sample was taken from Roger's Pass in the high, cold, snowcapped Selkirk Mountains of British Columbia, an area where the local Indians say the "snow spirit" lives. The setting is a high, rocky area laced with white-water streams. Winter snowfalls are tremendous here. To prevent serious avalanches, the highway patrols use large artillery guns to shoot down snowpacks before they get too big. When this road and the nearby train tunnel were built here, avalanches and sudden chilling storms killed a number of workmen.

Some of the reports for this sample were:

"I'm hearing a roaring like a waterfall or an ocean." (The sample was taken beside a rushing stream.)

"I'm looking at a stream with the banks rather sharply undercut." (Exactly correct!)

"I get the name Roger." (!)

"I'm feeling sacrifice, I think it's a human sacrifice." (Over two hundred lives were lost between 1885 and 1911 while the railroad was being constructed through this area.)

The next sample was collected in Ludington, Michigan, on the south side of Père Marquette Lake, just as it empties into Lake Michigan. The soil was taken from a sandy hill marked by a large, simple white cross marking the place where the Jesuit explorer Father Marquette died. From this tablespoon of soil, the group described the death of Father Marquette and his subsequent burial with the following reports:

"I'm picking up this sense of breathlessness, and I can hardly get sufficient breath to make comments. There's a tremendous stress or breathlessness."

"I'm feeling terrible, absolutely terrible, on the edge of nausea. I've been holding my head and thinking I'm not really dizzy, am I? It's a question of wooziness, sweaty palms, and cold feet."

"I'm lying down and can't get up. I'm feeling pain in my back. I'm alive but having a lot of trouble breathing."

"What I see is a very small shaft, like a mining shaft, and a man going down it headfirst."

Twenty-one of the twenty-seven reports on this soil sample follow these lines of a man getting sick and dying. It's hard to believe that they could have arrived at these impressions by chance.

The fifth sample was taken beside a downtown hotel in Sauk Centre, Minnesota. I chose this place because Sauk Centre is the birthplace of the well-known author Sinclair Lewis. Three quarters of the group's reports described a rural community, with lots of water, and land that had known periods of warming and cooling, that is, glaciation. No one picked up on Lewis, but the ambience of the place as well as its history came through, as people reported scenes of fields of wildflowers and an old cabin with a split-rail fence.

I gave a second set of the same samples to another Seattle sensitive, Robert Burdick, who did readings alone. He described two of the five places perfectly. For Roger's Pass, he described "Rocky area, at least six thousand feet elevation near a road or roadway, crystals nearby"—a 100 percent target hit.

In another replication of the same procedure with five samples of soil taken from around the Bay Area, sensitive Shelley Thompson also had several direct-target hits. For one sample collected at an Indian shell midden alongside San Francisco Bay, Thompson described an Indian village with fishing activity. Another sample was taken from the site of the old logging mill. Thompson's reading of this site described tall redwood trees with a small stream nearby and children playing. This is precisely what Old Mill Park in Mill Valley looks like today.

Soil seems to have a memory, which is somehow recorded holographically within the soil particles. People perceive the experience of place through physical sensations, visual imagery, and voices that come to them when in light trance states. They aren't 100 percent accurate in their readings but seem to do best when the history of a place is very emotional, as with the case of the site of Father Marquette's death or the mastodon massacre. Geomancers call this the predecessor factor and assert that it can be an important influence upon present-day life.

When Linda Juratovic of Four Dimensions Landscaping in Oakland, California, moved into a new office space, an old home, she and her partners were delighted. However, their secretary soon became ill and was ultimately diagnosed as having cancer. Her replacement was always late and was having a rough time keeping her love life together. On a whim, they moved her desk, and she began to feel better. However, the person who took her original place, Linda's boyfriend, Bob Thilgen, began to suffer deep depression. At this time Linda learned of the master Chinese geomancer Thomas Yun Lin and invited him over for a consultation. Master Lin made a number of suggestions and told Linda to check out who had previously owned the home and what had taken place in the various rooms. To her shock she found that the previous owner had died of cancer and that her bed was located exactly where the secretaries' and Bob's desk were. Master Lin did a complete geomantic cleaning, and soon the secretary had a new boyfriend and Bob's spirits cheered up considerably.

If you feel that you are occupying a space with a negative residual-memory problem, there are some things you can try that have been suggested to me by a number of geomantic wizards:

1. Fill the room with lighted white candles located in each of the corners of the room as well as in the middle. Let them burn for a while, while you burn some incense and play loud music. The idea is to fill the space with your vibrations.

2. If there is a particularly troubling spot, like the cancer desk in the Four Dimensions office, take a firecracker, put it in a big metal bowl, and place it on the floor in the middle of the place. Light the firecracker. The metal bowl will prevent the firecracker from starting a fire. The resulting boom will drive away anything negative, say the Chinese, who shoot off millions of firecrackers every year in San Francisco's Chinatown to drive away negative forces so that new, clean energies will enter their homes and businesses.

I know these suggestions will make some people laugh, but there are too many scientific data that support the conclusion that there are many more ways of perceiving than modern science says exist. Cultivating the subtle senses of perception has moved us to create the world's most spectacular architecture. All too often science tries to make the world fit existing theories rather than seeking better theories to explain what occurs.

DOWSING

Dowsing conventionally involves sensing the energies of the earth at a place. It can be done either on-site or at a distance using a map. Classically a person uses a forked stick made of hazel or willow to guide him or her to find underground water or metals. The dowser holds the wand in both hands and walks slowly with the third prong of the stick pointing forward. To activate the dowsing process, you think of what you're looking for, for example, underground water, a water pipe, iron ore, and so on. When you cross the "dowsing zone," the surface area above the underground target, the wand dips downward. Some dowsers can then go on and mentally ask questions about the depth of the water, its flow, and desirability. Modern dowsers often use a pendulum or a rod, which rotates around in a sleeve. These devices are what physicist William Tiller of Stanford University calls biomechanical transducers. They are amplifiers of personal sensations, that is, the instruments don't dowse, you do, and they simply record your dowsing reactions in the same way that muscle testing works.

In my workshops and classes over the past fifteen years, I've given hundreds of people dowsing wands. Over 80 percent have been delighted to find that they get dowsing reactions when walking over underground sprinkler pipes in a lawn, buried electrical wires, and sewer pipes. These results are in agreement with studies at Utah State and other universities sponsored by the U.S. Office of Water Resources Research. If you would like to try your hand at dowsing, the best source is the American Society of Dowsers in Danville, Vermont; ask for information about a local chapter.

In addition to locating domes and springs of water for new supplies, dowsers also assert that they can find negative earth energies, which can cause illness. "Pathogenic dowsing zones" are frequently associated with stagnant underground water. I was skeptical when I first heard this, but then an experience I had in Seattle made me reconsider.

In the spring of 1977, I moved into a lovely cottage on the west shore of Lake Washington, just north of Seattle. The setting was gorgeous, and it was an abnormally dry year. By November the winter rains began to fall. Shortly I developed arthritic pains in my legs, which grew worse and worse. A dowser came and dowsed the house and declared I was suffering from living over a pathogenic zone caused by rainwater collecting in a stagnant underground pool under the house. I was skeptical, but a physician wanted to give me cortisone shots, so instead we looked for another place to live. We moved to a new house near the university district, on high ground, and my pains disappeared in a couple of weeks.

The government of American Samoa includes units on parapsychology in its school curriculum. The Samoans teach the kids to think critically about psychic phenomena, but they also make it clear that thousands of years of living with a high dependency on psychic perception is not something you can discard as foolish superstition. Public-opinion polls find that three quarters of the population say they have had a psychic experience. Accepting and refining your psi abilities can be an important key to health and harmony with nature. On college campuses across the country you'll find psychology teachers insisting that dowsing is a hoax, while outside on the lawn the groundskeepers are at work with their wands locating the underground sprinkler pipes. Today, many oil and mining companies and even some major utility companies employ dowsers. Results should speak for themselves.

HARMONIZING WITH
THE SPIRIT OF PLACE

The term *geomancy* was first coined by Pliny the Elder in ancient Greece when he saw some Persian magi cast stones on the ground and then divine according to the patterns they saw. No one is quite sure where and when geomancy originated, but it's clear that one of its strongest roots comes from China, when the first emperor, Fu Hsi, looked upward and identified symbols and images in the stars. Then he looked to the earth and observed patterns in nature. From these initial observations eventually arose the *I Ching,* which interprets these patterns as both an oracle and a book of wisdom. One of the applications of the *I Ching* is its use to create an octagonal symbol called the *ba-gua,* which is used by Chinese geomancers to determine how directions influence the *chi* of each place.

Modern Western science still has trouble with the concept of a life-force energy, *chi*, but acupuncture is now licensed as a legitimate health-care approach in most states. Acupuncture works by manipulating *chi* with needles, massage, and the burning of an herb called *moxa*, which is placed over special places on the body. The wisdom of ancient China also asserts that the *chi* of the earth can also be manipulated. Those who work with the *chi* of nature and in design practice the art and science of *feng shui*, which translates literally as "wind and water," implying that this approach to landscape design and architecture works with natural energy flows to aid health, wealth, and creativity.

One of the most popular speakers at the "Spirit of Place" symposiums has been Thomas Yun Lin, the grand master of Black Sect Tantric Buddhism for the world and an internationally recognized *feng shui* geomancer. Master Lin's temple is in Berkeley, California, located on the crest of a hill on Russell Street, a tree-lined artery that climbs from San Francisco Bay to the Berkeley hills. From the outside the temple is a four-story gray mansion with a surrounding yard decorated with appealing shrubs, rocks, birdbath, and gently flowing pools of water. The first hint that something special is going on inside is the bright-red door.

When you enter, the first sight you see is a wall of mirrors behind the door, absorbing any incoming negative energies and reflecting back blessings on those who enter with positive energy. Stepping inside the door, your mind expects to see a living room and dining room. Instead you are greeted by massive altars filled with statues of Buddha and other deities, icons, burning candles, and the pungent aroma of incense. The windows are covered by shades, and the light of the candles and the aromas quickly put your mind in a reverent mood.

A staircase in the center of the house sends a brilliant shaft of light penetrating the heavy decorum of the first floor. The light streams in from windows and a skylight above and is reflected by numerous mirrors on the walls of the ascending stairs. If the house is a symbol of self, as architect Clare Cooper Marcus has proposed, then clearly this home is the residence of an enlightened holy man.

A jolly, bearlike man with a captivating smile and a bubbly personality, Master Lin was described by one television reporter as a "Chinese Buddy Hackett." While his manner is nearly always cheerful, his work with *feng shui* is deadly serious. Recently Master Lin has lectured at the United Nations, consulted on interior design for the I. M. Pei–designed offices of Creative Artists Agency in Los Angeles, worked with corporate clients such as the Bank of Hong Kong, and had personal meetings with the Dalai Lama, Pope John Paul, and President George Bush.

In Master Lin's view *feng shui* seeks to adjust the *chi* in and around each person so that they will be healthy, happy, and prosperous. He says there are three kinds of *chi:* one that circulates in the earth, one that circulates in the atmosphere, and a third that moves through our bodies. Successful *feng shui* comes from aligning these three forms of *chi* with the Tao, the life force of nature that arises from the continuous interplay of yin and yang.

One of Master Lin's favorite Chinese sayings is,

Being born with good looks is not as important as being born with a good fate or destiny.

Being born with a good fate or destiny is not as important as having a kind heart.

Having a kind heart is not as important as having a positive state of *chi.*

To maximize positive *chi* in a person's life, *feng shui* works with two interrelated systems. *Sying,* the art of forms, is similar to landscape architecture and interior design. A steep-rising hill has a certain kind of *chi,* just as a dismal swamp has a negative feeling. The *chi* of a place creates a mood and draws the spirits that are attracted to the *chi.* Master Lin's temple is located at the head of a "dragon line" whose tail begins at San Francisco Bay. Lin says that the heaviness of the first floor in the temple is purposeful, to ground the dragon's uprising energy and transform it from materiality to spirituality. Other land forms and their associated spirits may be seen as tigers, lions, snakes, elephants, turtles, rams, and boars, which are also found in the Chinese astrological system. Striking harmonies between forms on the land and those in the sky is an essential part of *feng shui*'s work in landscape design and is a view shared by most other kinds of geomancy of the world as well.

The art of working with *sying* is called *ru-shr* and involves the art of placement. A wind chime tinkling in the breeze attracts positive *chi.* Uplifted-form trees, such as Lombardy poplars, cause the *chi* of a place to rise, whereas low shrubs, such as junipers, ground it. Flagpoles and lights on poles can raise the spirits of a place, making it feel happier.

Once the outside *chi* has been properly cultivated, it is guided into a home, and the main entry door to each room is its "mouth of the *chi.*" A mirror placed opposite the door helps drive away negative energies and blesses those who enter with good intentions.

According to Black Sect Tantric Buddist teachings, the best *feng shui* results arise from placements that follow an eight-sided ancient Chinese diagram called the *ba-gua,* an esoteric explanation of the compass which ascribes certain powers to each direction. According to Master Lin's *ba-gua,* the north, for example, is the direction of career and is harmonious with water and the color black. The west is harmonious with the element metal, the color white, and children. The south is harmonious with fire and the color red, as well as fame. The east is harmonious with the element wood, the color green, the family, and so on. In an exterior setting, starting from scratch, you can use these colors and directions as they are, but if you have an existing home or room, Master Lin advises that the main doorway to the home or room be considered the "mouth of the *chi*" and the *ba-gua* for that room use that entrance as north regardless of what the actual direction is. The idea here is that making an adjustment in a corner of a room corresponding to an aspect of a person's life will influence the course of affairs for the people who use that space. To fully appreciate the *ba-gua* and its use in *feng shui* you should take some time to familiarize yourself with Chinese philosophy and consult one of the several books written about *feng shui.*

Some of the simple *ru-shr* cures to improve the *chi* of a home or office include the following:

1. Install bright objects, mirrors, and crystal balls in open spaces and opposite doors to deflect bad *chi* and to brighten up spaces. The general rule is the bigger the better. Lights can also help make *chi* more positive, especially upturned lights.
2. Install bells or wind chimes that make pleasant sounds. These dispel negative *chi* and summon positive *chi.*
3. Cultivate living objects around your home—plants, fishbowls, flowers, bird feeders, or birdbaths.
4. Place heavy objects such as stones or statues in places to help stabilize energy, such as beneath a typewriter or computer or beside an entryway.
5. Install moving objects—mobiles, windmills, and fountains—all of which stimulate healthy *chi* flow.
6. Bamboo flutes can be used for decoration or played. They symbolize spiritual swords, and tying red ribbons around them and pointing them upward helps elevate *chi* flow. Shaking flutes helps drive away negative energies and spirits.
7. Place machines powered by electricity in special places according to *ba-gua* design.
8. Choose colors to increase beneficial *chi.* Yellow is the Chinese color of longevity, red is an auspicious color, and green is a color of spring and growth.
9. Red ribbons can be placed on doors with knocking knobs, fringe can be used to hide slanting beams, and so on.

10. Always place a bed or desk so that it is in the corner of the room opposite the door, facing the door. If you have your back to a door, you will feel uneasy. If you are directly facing the door, the incoming *chi* may be too upsetting, and you may have too much stress and be unable to relax or concentrate on your work.

Ru-shr is effective, but Master Lin says that implementing design changes alone will result in only 10- to 20-percent potential results. To have *feng shui* produce really good results, you must also use *chu-shr*. The transcendental cure for the second element of *feng shui* is *yi*, which means "will, wish, and intention." *Yi* is a blessing and is a state of mind that is used as you implement the *ru-shr* adjustments. To obtain the best results you should make *ru-shr* adjustments with *chu-shr* intentions of good *yi*.

Chu-shr works with prayer, visualizations, and gestures called mudras and often involves simple rituals. If you are having a problem with your work, for example, a *chu-shr* approach might be to light a candle at the career place in your office, say some prayers, and visualize yourself becoming successful. A *feng shui* strategy for settling a household quarrel might be to burn some incense in the family position and think of peace and harmony rather than arguing.

Chu-shr requires time, patience, and self-development, but according to Master Lin it is almost always 100-percent successful. If you would like to learn more about *feng shui*, there are two good books written about Master Lin's Black Sect Tantric Buddhist approach, both by Sarah Rossbach. They are *Feng Shui: The Chinese Art of Placement* and *Interior Design with Feng Shui.*

Consulting with
the Spirit of Place

I'll let you decide if nature spirits are discarnate entities or symbolic interpretations of the spirit of a place. But keep in mind that in Iceland, if an environmental-impact statement claims that a stone, a grove of trees, or a hill is the home of *huldrafolk,* "elves," developers will avoid disturbing the place.

To consult with the spirit of a place, whether in person or at a distance, many people have found the following imagery exercise useful. If you are on-site at the place, before you do this journey, walk the land slowly. Place some cornmeal beside a tree as a way of showing respect. As you explore the land, find some edible plants and chew on them—dandelions and plantain are almost everywhere. If there is a well, drink some water. If it's morning, look for some dew on the grass to moisten your tongue.

Now find a quiet place where you can lie down and not be disturbed for half an hour. Again, if you are at the site itself, lie directly on the earth. If you are at a distance and you have a stone or some other object from the place you want to study, hold it in your hand.

At first most people find it useful to have some background music or the rhythm of a drum or rattle, plus a voice guiding them along. After you have practiced this for a time, you can just slip into this reverie without any help.

The Spirit-of-Place Journey

Relax in a comfortable place where you will not be disturbed for up to half an hour. Since you will be exploring a place on the earth and its meaning to you, the best results seem to come when you are lying on the earth directly.

Begin your journey by closing your eyes and taking in several deep breaths and letting them out slowly, making a sound if you like. Now think of a place you would like to explore and understand better. It could be the place where you are or it could be one some distance away. In your mind's eye see this place as vividly as possible. Try to attune your mind to the place, and when you feel a harmony has been reached, hum what you feel is the rhythm and feel of that place. Do this for half a minute or so.

Now see yourself in this place. The more vividly you can picture yourself there, the better. Feel the sun or wind. Smell the odors. Feel the ground under your feet. Get to know the place.

Now clap your hands together, and as you clap them, a magical staff appears in your hands. This is a staff of power, your own personal earth-wisdom symbol. Examine the staff. What is it made of? Does it have any special carvings or decorations? This is an instrument of power. Later you may want to make a staff like this.

Now take the staff into your right hand. Raise the staff into the air and strike it down on the ground, and as you do, you will find yourself wearing a special suit of clothes. Examine these clothes. They represent your earth-wisdom costume. You may want to make or buy something like this later on as well.

With your staff and special earth-wisdom suit on, look all around you, moving in a 360-degree circle. Upon completing this survey of the land, raise your staff into the air and strike it down on the ground. Now ask that the spirit of this place come forward. Again, circle slowly, looking for something new and different. It could be an animal, a cloud, an unusual-shaped "spirit," or a familiar cat or dog. This is a voice for the place. Ask it questions. See what it can tell you. Perhaps it may want to take you someplace to see something. This is a guide for understanding this place.

Take as long as you like to explore this place with your guide.

When you have completed your journey, thank your guide. You can return again anytime you'd like. Now thank the place.

Now raise your staff again and strike it on the ground. This time your costume and staff will disappear, and the place will fade away.

Become aware of your body and the ground underneath you. Open your eyes.

After you have finished this exercise, draw a picture of the spirit you found. Some people find that if they put this picture in a place and meditate on it, it seems to "talk" to them. You could say that it simply continues the work of seeing in the mind's eye with creative imagery, or you could say that it works by sympathetic magic to keep you attuned to your place of power.

I've used this exercise with hundreds of people, ranging from elementary school–age children to professional architects and planners, with many startling results. A related procedure can be used to see if your dreams can help you come to a better understanding of a place. Before going to sleep at night, eat some plant life from the place you are at and drink some water if possible. Lay your sleeping bag directly on the ground. You may want to light a candle or say some prayers asking for guidance from the place. Using this method, I've sometimes had dreams about the history of a place that have proven especially interesting for deciphering the meaning of petroglyphs or archeological artifacts.

Your dreams may also shed light on land-use controversies. I was asked by a newly formed institute to do a geomantic reading of their land. After walking the land, that night in my dreams I saw myself lying in bed and heard heavy footsteps at the door. I felt a sense of fear and dread and remembered that a mirror was placed opposite the door. Just as I thought this, the door opened, and a man in a white sheet looking like a member of the Ku Klux Klan entered the room. He stopped short as he saw the mirror. The next day, upon questioning my hosts, I discovered that they had received threatening letters from some people in the area who were afraid their institute might be corrupting the community. The spirit of a place is the result of the interplay between the spiritual world and nature, and the collective product of the interactions of the people of that area too. When they all come into harmony, the spirit of place can really work its magic best.

Translating the Spirit of Place into Art and Action

Places move us, and the mind is a symbolizer. Spirit-of-place art offers some of the world's most inspiring examples of mind and nature in harmony. In Seattle, Washington, a group of architects and designers called the Geo Group are at work energizing the spirit of Seattle with public art located at "power points" in the city, and their work is being funded by the city Arts Commission. Their approach is to use dowsing to map out the city's places of power. Then they draw connecting lines, which they call ley lines, and where the lines intersect exist what the Geo Group calls places of power. They then use this information to site public art that evokes the spirit of that place and that radiates its powers outward to inspire people. Like the Druids of England in approach, the group is getting lots of support for an idea that one hopes will catch on in other American cities that are suffering from a lack of identity.[4]

On a larger scale, the Bioregional Movement in the United States seeks to encourage people to pay less attention to their political boundaries and more to geographic land forms to grow a local, unique culture from the resources at hand. The rationale is that when people lose touch with the place where they live as an ecological entity, their ability to live in harmony with nature decreases.

For example, I live in the Shasta Bioregion, which has low coastal mountains, elevations under five thousand feet above sea level, a temperate woodland natural ecosystem, and lots of fog and water at certain times of the year. If you'd like to find out more about bioregionalism and the bioregion where you live, write to New Options, P.O. Box 19324, Washington, D.C. 20036, for a great bioregional map, which costs about two dollars. Another good place to find out about bioregionalism, "reinhabiting the earth," as Peter Berg and Ray Dasmann put it, is the Planet Drum Foundation, Box 31251, San Francisco, CA 94131.

Chapter Eight

PERSONAL POWER
AND NATURE

*Wherever I found the living,
there I found the will
to power.*

—FRIEDRICH NIETZSCHE
Thus Spake Zarathustra

During his fifty-three-year career as a horticulturist, Luther Burbank produced more than 800 new plants, which today have given us new varieties of potatoes, prunes, walnuts, apples, peaches, tomatoes, the Shasta daisy, and many more, including more than 25 marketable vegetables and 250 salable fruits. Until his death in 1926 people from all over the world flocked to see him and his gardens, including Thomas Edison, Henry Ford, Helen Keller, Jack London, John Muir, John Burroughs, and the king and queen of Belgium.

Burbank had little formal training, but he understood how to breed and propagate plants like no one else. One apple tree in his orchard had 526 varieties of apples on its branches, and a nearby cherry tree had more than 400 kinds of cherries.

One of Burbank's most astounding creations was a spineless variety of prickly pear cactus, designed to create food for cattle in arid areas. When Burbank was visited by the Indian holy man Yogananda, the swami declared him a saint. So moved was Burbank by the blessing that he confessed to Yogananda that he had created the spineless cactus not by science but by talking to the plant. He simply said that he gave the plant love and told it it didn't need its spines for protection. At his home in Santa Rosa several of his spineless cactus plants still grow. A number of the pads or leaves of the cactus are heart-shaped, which I do not find in other spineless cactuses with such frequency. Burbank believed that part of his success was due to living in Santa Rosa, California, which he said "is the chosen spot of all the earth as far as Nature is concerned."

Luther Burbank understood plants out of his sensitive awareness of their souls and he knew how to make things happen that no one else could. He was a man of personal power, something we all yearn for. Personal power has many forms, and a common element among the lives of truly powerful people is an intimate connection with nature.

"The greatest delight which the fields and woods minister is the suggestion of an occult relationship between man and the vegetable," Ralph Waldo Emerson proclaimed in 1846. Another man who rose to world eminence through his ability to perceive nature was Rudolf Steiner, who developed agricultural techniques to strengthen soil through composting and special labor-intensive cultivation methods. A mystical philosopher, scientist, and educator who lived from 1861 to 1925, Steiner built his whole life on developing abilities to see into the heart of things. He agreed with Aristotle about man's essential sympathies with nature, asserting that "man has his physical body with the minerals, his ether body with the plants, . . . and his astral body of the same nature as the animals."[1]

Steiner was practicing the "new physics" sixty years before anyone else. "If we enter deeply into the nature of the living world," he believed, "we naturally begin to create in such a way that what we apprehend inwardly in the spirit can take on the most manifold outward forms."[2]

Today, nearly seven decades after his passing, the world is just beginning to appreciate Steiner's gifts, including biodynamic gardening, the Waldorf education method, eurythmic exercises, natural philosophy, and organic architecture. One of the greatest indications of Steiner's power is that Adolf Hitler, one of the more powerful people of the twentieth century, considered Steiner the most dangerous person alive, and unsuccessfully tried on several occasions to have him killed. Hitler feared Steiner, for he felt that regardless of what he did, Steiner could read his every move through his remarkable intuitive powers.

My dictionary lists thirteen different definitions for *power;* most of them involve gaining control over something or making something happen. Scholars say that "knowledge is power." "Money is power," insist business-minded people. The lyrics of rock-and-roll songs and ads in magazines say, "Sex is power." Power comes in many forms. Feeling powerless is one of the most common of all human complaints today, which indicates that the methods of gaining power are not well understood.

Power is a measure of our ability to get the things we want, and "it is the desire for power that keeps most people working," Michael Korda proposes in his important book, *Power: How to Get It, How to Use It.* Most human conflicts involve power struggles. A first step to increasing personal power is to clarify the workings of what psychiatrist Alfred Adler believed to be among the most central of human drives—the will to gain power.

SPORTS AND PERSONAL POWER

In the early 1970s Michael Murphy, founder of the Esalen Institute in California, and a number of other explorers of human potentiality teamed up to study the secrets of peak performance in sports. I joined the team and worked with distance runner Mike Spino to produce a large symposium held in Eugene, Oregon, in 1975, "Exploring the Human Potential Through Physical Activity: Body, Mind and Spirit." The program featured many of the leaders of the human-potential movement holding seminars with members of the Professional Track Association over a week-long period that culminated in a pro track meet seen by a crowd of five thousand. A common goal of both the humanists and some of the world's best athletes was to better understand how personal power works.

A synthesis of the work of the Esalen Sports Center is reported in an extraordinary book, *The Psychic Side of Sports,* by Murphy and Rhea White, which distills the stories of more than 4,500 athletes talking about moments of peak performance in all kinds of sports. What emerges from this exhaustive study of the psychology of extraordinary sports performance is that more strain doesn't necessarily mean more gain. The key to powerful performance is closely related to mental concentration, clarity of intention, and proper attitude—providing one's body is physically fit.

According to Michael Murphy, the mental state of the athlete engaged in a period of unusually powerful performance is characterized by certain common elements:

1. Extraordinary perceptual clarity—sights, sounds, odors, and physical sensations seem to become clearer and distinct in a way not normally experienced in everyday life
2. Concentration that becomes very focused, like the one-pointedness of mind the Zen meditator seeks to achieve
3. A sense of emptiness and feeling of unity that seem to envelop the field of play, resulting in the feeling that time itself has slowed down and that one's actions have become an expression of merger with a higher force or purpose
4. Access to new energies, which fill one's mind and body, moving one to new and more profound levels of inspiration and vitality
5. As a result of all of the above, experiences that are called paranormal, such as telepathy, clairvoyance, precognition, psychokinesis, auric vision, and unusual physical strength, become normal[3]

This research, which was very controversial when released in the mainstream sports community, has become a prime force in the use of relaxation techniques, martial arts, yoga, mental imagery, and self-hypnosis programs by nearly all professional and college teams today.

The lessons from studies of peak performance in sports appear to have relevance for becoming more powerful in other aspects of life. Mental-training systems such as those previously mentioned help one gain control over what psychologist Charles Tart considers the three mental barriers to increasing personal power:

1. Loading—keeping one's mind busy with "chatter" when it should be concentrating.
2. Feedback—Negative feedback about one's behavior or one's potential to accomplish certain things results in inhibited behaviors and a negative attitude about life that breeds resentment and jealousy. Positive feedback, on the other hand, helps shape better and better performance. Critical thinking is important, of course, but it should be directed toward how to do things better next time, not how bad things were this time.
3. Limiting beliefs—self-censorship to avoid emotionally charged areas of life prevents many aspects of growth and the expression of personal power.[4]

SUGGESTION: The symbols that move us are an expression of our individual nature, which is the source of all true power. If you were able to make a mythical animal of power that would be most potent to you, what would it look like? For example, such a creature might have the legs and body of a deer for speed, the wings of an eagle to fly high above things for perspective, and the head of an owl for wisdom. Try creating your own special mythic power animal in a drawing. Make up a story or a poem about what life for this creature might be like. Forms like this often became translated into ritual, crests, and even landscape forms, such as the strange giant animals that dot the Nazca plains of Peru or the Serpent Mound of Ohio.

LEVELS OF POWER

Not all power is the same. There are degrees of power, like gears in a car, that seem to occur in a sequence.

LEVEL 1: FOCUSED CONCENTRATION AND INTENTION

Level 1 involves focused concentration and dedication to your effort, which leads to one-pointedness of mind and action. Coupled with the right inspiration and discipline, a person can learn to slip more frequently into what Bob Kriegel calls "the zone"— that space from which prowess flows with seemingly less and less effort whether you're playing chess, picking a melody on your guitar, or shooting an arrow at a target.

The more power one exerts in the world, the more changes become possible, and the more responsibility for those changes one takes on. Some of the most common techniques for developing personal power are visualizing yourself as being powerful and successful and making positive, affirmative statements that you will be powerful. Thoughts carry intentions. Positive thinking helps as long as you use it correctly. But realize that other people also get their wishes. Several years ago some people in Oregon located a man who seemed like he might give money for a holistic birth center they were trying to start. Prior to an important meeting with him, to try to make the deal go through, the group met and visualized him giving them money while chanting that he would do so. When they arrived at his house for the meeting about the gift, he was being taken into a waiting ambulance. It seemed that he had just had a heart attack.

Rev. Olga Worrall told me that when you pray, you should

always give people the option of not receiving your thoughts. Her prayer for health was to hold a picture of someone in her mind and say, "May so-and-so be united with God, *if they so choose to be.*" Working with power, the most important thing is to not force the universe. Follow Confucius' wisdom: Heaven directs things, the earth produces, and man cooperates to create success.

LEVEL 2: SURRENDERING EGO

Level-2 power kicks in when control lessens and surrender becomes more important. The ego boundaries that got you to Level 1 somehow dissolve, and you unite with the larger reality around you, feeling an unusual oneness with nature that in turn seems to become a force driving you. World-class distance runner Ken Foreman described his experience in setting a world-record distance time: "That day was magic. Once the starter's gun went off, I seemed to slip into an almost dreamlike state. I don't remember my feet touching the ground. I just sort of blended into nature, and by the time I realized what was happening, I had broken the tape with my fastest time ever."

Sports psychologists call Foreman's peak performance moment a flow experience. A similar flow experience ignited the life of David Smith while he was swimming across Golden Gate Strait. In high school Smith had been a champion swimmer, but after being thrown out of college twice he had given up on sports to become a bar owner, an acknowledged leader of the "good life" in San Francisco. In his autobiography, *Healing Journey: The Odyssey of an Uncommon Athlete,* Smith tells how one afternoon while parked with a girlfriend watching the sun paint pictures on the fog and riptides of the Golden Gate, he suddenly felt a calling to swim the Gate. After several months of arduous training, he waded into the icy waters, took the plunge, and made an unexpected discovery.

"Almost immediately an odd thing happened to me. Just after

I got into the water, my body felt possessed by a strange sensation as if tiny charges of electricity were running through the nerve endings. At first I attributed it to excitement . . . but the feeling was different from any high or excitement I had experienced before. It flowed through me like a powerful guidance system."

As Smith tore through treacherous tides, ancient Greek myths came to mind, and he recalled images of the fire that burns inside man's soul when he is in alignment with the life force. Inspired by this experience, he went on to set the world's record for the twenty-four-hour nonstop indoor swim—forty-one miles! And that was just the beginning. Soon he swam sixty-three miles down the Sacramento River and thirty miles down the icy-cold Russian River. Each time as he slipped into the water and began his rhythm, a force possessed him. Taking on a bigger challenge, he swam across the Strait of Gibraltar from Africa to Europe—the first time it had ever been done.

Smith says his extraordinary feats arise from blending with "the source." "When there is accord between man and nature," he says, "between self and place, then there is contact with the source."

The sense of unity of mind, body, and spirit with nature that Smith refers to is the mind-set from which feats of extraordinary powers may arise. One of the most dramatic examples of how ego surrender aids in the performance of unusual physical feats is fire walking, an ancient ritual act now widely taught as a pathway to personal growth by transcending fear. Thousands of participants who have gone through a three-hour preparatory ritual with Tolly Burkan, Larissa Valenskaya, and other teachers of this remarkable practice seldom develop blisters walking barefoot across the pit, even though the coals are at least 1,200 degrees Fahrenheit. According to Dr. Bruce Achauer of the University of California at Irvine Medical Center, flesh should burn almost instantly at that temperature, and yet if people are

in the right state of mind—a nonjudgmental trusting of spirit—
their feet simply don't burn![5]

The sweat lodge, a traditional healing and purification technique described in an earlier chapter, can also be a tool to help
people discover and more fully express their personal power.
"What a 'sweat' does is help you to let go of your distractions
and fears and tap into universal wisdom, which then becomes a
vital force to help you surrender to who you really are," asserts
movie and television actor Max Gail, known to millions for his
portrayal of the lovable cop "Wojo" on the *Barney Miller* television series. A strong supporter of Indian rights, Max's work with
native peoples has led him to a deeper understanding of the
nature kingdom through encounters with their spiritual life. Max
feels that the tapestry of natural elements woven into the sweat
lodge, a ritual form which is found all around the world in
circumpolar peoples, is a valuable natural process that can enable
people to achieve the clarity of mind and inspiration essential for
vital artistic expression.

LEVEL 3: ADDING THE POWER OF PLACE

Australian aborigines have been known to track a wounded
kangaroo for eighty miles. Masai hunters in East Africa may
chase antelope a similar distance, simply running their prey to
exhaustion. Among the Hopi, Zuñi, and Papago Indians of the
American Southwest, distance running is a part of traditional
religious ceremonies. In the Papago salt journey, men run four
days each way to the ocean to gather salt. They must run
carefully, not offending any animals whose spirits would cause
bad fortune. Each night they must sleep with their head toward
the ocean "so that its power can draw them on." At least one day
they must run without any water and on the way home they
must be silent and no one can touch their bodies.

Right alignments with nature are a very pure source of power.

Chief Letakots-Lesa of the Pawnee told researcher Natalie Curtis in 1904, "In the beginning of all things, wisdom and knowledge were with the animals; for Tirawa, the One Above, did not speak directly to man. He sent certain animals to tell men that he showed himself through the beasts, and that from them, and from the stars and the sun and the moon, man should learn. Tirawa spoke to man through his works."[6]

The Tarajumara Indians of Mexico undertake a thirty- to forty-mile cross-country running race called the *rarapira* in which teams of men or women run barefoot while kicking a wooden ball carved from the root of a juniper tree. When invited to join in the Olympics, the Tarajumaras complained that the distances are too short.

To the Lum Gom runners, the priest messengers of the mountains of Tibet, the distances of the Tarajumaras are warm-ups. After a long period of training that works on concentration more than physical conditioning, the Lum Goms are rumored to be able to run for days without stopping. The key to doing this, of course, is to learn to master a trance state, where they remain tapped into the source very powerfully and then draw power from the places they pass through.

"There are mountains which are just mountains and there are mountains with personality," observed Lama Anagarika Govinda. "Personality consists in the power to influence others, and this power is due to consistency, harmony and one-pointedness of character. If these qualities are present in an individual in their highest perfection, he is a fit leader for humanity, be he a ruler, a thinker or a saint; and we recognize him as a vessel of supramundane power. If these qualities are present in a mountain, we recognize it as a vessel of cosmic power and we call it a sacred mountain."[7]

Personal power is a state of extreme self-expression. As mind-body unity is achieved, more power results from reaching out to form right alignments and identification with nature. To call a spade a spade, this book is a training manual in wizardry. The path to acquiring power requires learning to work with natural energies and powers.

One of the most important teachers of extraordinary powers of our time is Carlos Castaneda, whose writing describes his growing understanding of the world of sorcery through association with various people of power. In *Journey to Ixtlan,* Castaneda described a time when his teacher, Don Juan, introduced him to the importance of place in becoming powerful:

> Fix all this in your memory. This spot is yours. This morning you *saw,* and that was the omen. You found this spot by *seeing.* The omen was unexpected, but it happened. You are going to hunt power whether you like it or not. It is not a human decision, not yours or mine. Now properly speaking, this hilltop is your place, your beloved place; all that is around you is under your care. You must look after everything here and everything will in turn look after you.[8]

In support of Don Juan's guidance is the ancient Irish belief that a chief is married to a special place, which becomes both a wife and a mother to the chief. The name for both these special places and the chiefs is *tuath.*

At the 1989 "Spirit of Place" symposium Vine Deloria, Jr., described the psychic connection between people and place as so important to power and mental health that "unless the sacred places are discovered and protected and used as religious places, there is no possibility of a nation ever coming to grips with the land itself and national psychic stability is impossible."

SUGGESTION: According to *feng shui* geomancy, the most powerful place in any room is the corner diagonal to the door. The least powerful position is to have your back facing the door. Try sitting in each of these positions and see how you feel. The next time you go out to a restaurant, experiment with sitting at tables in these positions to see how you feel. Cultivate your ability to see and sense the most powerful places indoors and outdoors.

Powerful Places

All around the world, and for nearly all of human history until modern times, there have been certain special caves, valleys, mountains, groves, stones, and springs—"hierophonies," according to Mircea Eliade—which have been declared sacred because they seem to manifest a power that helps people slip into states in which extraordinary events, "krakophanies," occur. Eliade had no doubt about the existence of sacred places as specific sites of power, for he writes:

> The rocks, springs, caves and woods venerated from the earliest historic times are still, in different forms, held as sacred by Christian communities today. A superficial observer might well see this aspect of popular piety as a "superstition," and see in it proof that all community religious life is largely made up of things inherited from prehistoric times. But what the continuity of the sacred places in fact indicates is the autonomy of hierophonies; the sacred expresses itself according to laws of its own dialectic and this expression comes to man *from without.* If the *choice* of his sacred places were left to man himself, then there could be no explanation for this continuity.[9]

To better understand how the power of place affects people, for the last decade I have been collecting stories of unusual experiences associated with special places. The more than two hundred stories reviewed to date have come from biographies of famous people, such as Carl Jung, Rachel Carson, and Gifford Pinchot, as well as from people I have seen in therapy, those who have told their stories to me in person, and others who have written to me. In analyzing the data, I have set aside experiences of people who were under the influence of hallucinogenic drugs, since their states of consciousness were influenced by the chemicals. My conclusion is that place plays a crucial role in making the experience happen. It both helps the boundaries between the worlds to dissolve and allows the sacred dimension of life to show itself. Such experiences tend to have the following characteristics:

1. The experience usually begins with a feeling of being drawn to a place for no apparent reason.
2. Once people arrive, they sense an "extra energy" and possibly see unusual animal behavior.
3. A sight or sound often seems to trigger a new state of consciousness in which the normal ego boundaries slip away. According to Marghanita Laski, experiences of ecstasy take place "almost always after contact with something valuable or beautiful, or both."[10]
4. A new sense of energy floods the person, and with it come perceptual changes: Time slows down, the world takes on an exceptional clarity, and it seems as though the symbolic and mythic dimensions of life become more clear and present.
5. There is usually an experience of mental-emotional unity that cannot fully be put into words, which is then followed by some type of manifestation of unusual powers.
6. The entire experience seldom lasts over half an hour, although the energizing effects may last for hours or days.
7. Forever after, your life is changed, and you feel a deeper, richer sense of nature and a desire to protect it. Radical Catholic theologian Matthew Fox has observed, "A moment of ecological awakening is also a moment of spiritual awakening, and vice versa." Transcendental experiences in nature appear to be a fundamental aspect of human nature with tremendous relevance to personal and cultural survival.

VARIETIES OF TRANSPERSONAL EXPERIENCES
ASSOCIATED WITH SPECIAL PLACES

I must be distantly related to Linnaeus, because to understand sacred experiences, I've created a taxonomy. Each experience is unique, of course, and some may contain more than one element of this taxonomy, but this at least helps us understand the range of possibilities when we connect ourselves with a sacred place and the gods are with us.

1. Unitive Bonding with Nature and Special Places

When actor-activist Robert Redford was ten years old, recovering from a mild case of polio, his mother took him to Yosemite National Park. Redford was swept up in the splendor of the valley. "I said to myself, 'That's it—I want to be a part of that.' I started right then. I spent more time outdoors. I started to hike. I went to Yosemite to work, and I learned to climb there."[11]

John Muir had a similar attraction for Yosemite, as have many others, but a place need not be massive to evoke special feelings. William Stapp, former director of environmental education for UNESCO, traces his lifelong commitment to conservation to an experience he had while studying a tide pool as a college freshman. Somehow the beauty and intricacies of life in that tiny pocket of water moved him to realize that everything is connected to everything else. The rapture was so great, he almost drowned in the incoming tide.

2. Feelings of Bliss, Awe, and Wonder

Eco-poet-laureate Gary Snyder wrote in his book *The Old Ways* about his childhood in Washington State, of growing up in the "ghost of an old-growth forest": "When I was young, I had an immediate, deep sympathy with the natural world . . . an undefinable awe. An attitude of gratitude, wonder and a sense of protection, especially as I began to see the hills being bulldozed for roads, and the forests of the Pacific Northwest magically float away on logging trucks."[12]

Carl Jung reported that while standing on Mount Kilimanjaro in Africa and looking across the plains teeming with wild game, he saw himself as part of the ongoing pageant of life, a link in the continuing evolutionary chain connecting past, present, and future. This perception forever after gave his life a sense of perspective, showing him his place in history.

3. Waking Visions

In the spring of 1652 George Fox climbed atop Pendle Hill in Lancashire, England, and received a vision of a "great people to be gathered." The result was the formation of the Quaker religion. In a similar experience in New York State in 1830, Joseph Smith had a vision while exploring an Indian mound. This led to his founding the Mormon religion. In the Bible (Luke 4:5) Jesus is described as climbing a high mountain, led by the devil. Reaching the summit "in a moment of time," he was shown all the kingdoms of the world. In a similar fashion Muhammad had visions and heard voices on Mount Ararat, and Moses and Elijah spoke with God on Horeb.

4. Interspecies Communication and Cooperation

Visiting Shark and Turtle Rock, a very sacred place in American Samoa, I made a simple prayer and tossed some food into the sea. Legend has it that a shark and a turtle are supposed to come to the surface here and swim in a circle for five minutes or so when children of the nearby village of Vaitogi sing the correct chant. In response to my gesture of respect, a whale breached just offshore and frolicked for about five minutes.

A woman reported how she had felt depressed and went for a drive, ending up at a deserted forest campground. She got out and was greeted by a blue jay that landed on a picnic table and coaxed her to follow as it hopped along a trail. She did and soon found herself looking at the spellbinding view of Mount Hood. Tears welled up in her eyes, and she felt a profound wave of bliss flow through her. In a few minutes it passed. The jay hopped down from a tree and led her back to her car. She got in and drove away, her depression lifted.

5. Vivid Dreams

Carl Jung suggested that people visiting certain places would have dreams and visions containing the same symbols and mythic themes. He called this "psychic localization." Many people visiting Indian Hot Springs in West Texas report having vivid dreams of tall, nearly naked Indians and bands of wild horses.

In Australia aborigines go on "dream treks," during which they walk cross-country in a ritual, stopping to spend the night at certain places where they hope they will have special dreams. In the hills above Santa Barbara, California, the Chumash Indians used special caves for seeking dreams. The symbols of their visions remain painted on the walls of some of the caves.

My colleague, anthropologist Lisa Faithorn, went on a pilgrimage to the sacred places of India. One day she journeyed to an area where the rain forest had been clear-cut on a sacred mountain. That night she had a dream about the trees crying. She has since started a whole new teaching program about spiritual ecology.

6. Hearing Unusual Sounds and Smelling Unusual Odors

Hiking on Mount Shasta, writer Patricia Kollings heard strange tinkling noises. A friend told her that these were spirit bells of the mountain, which others have reported hearing there. That night Kollings had a vivid dream showing the fiery volcanic bowels of the mountain, and she got up and wrote pages of moving poetry.

On holiday visiting the island of Iona, off the coast of Scotland, a couple reported smelling flowers in the air where none were to be seen. They later found out that such flowers were used in certain old religious ceremonies that used to be conducted on this special island.

7. Ancestral-Memory Recollections

Visiting the ruins on Mount Olympus, the well-known sensitive Anne Armstrong felt intense sexual feelings pulsating in her

body. She later found that she had been in an area where Diony-
sian rites had once been held.

Visiting Chaco Canyon, author Eleanor Gadon tried and tried
to understand the petroglyphs she saw on the canyon walls but
could find no one to help her. That night in a dream an Indian
woman came and told her what they meant.

Walking the trails of his ancestors on Bodega Head along the
Pacific Ocean, Kashia Pomo Indian Lorin Smith heard "voices"
from his ancestors calling to him. Soon, through dreams, he
received instructions on how to build a ceremonial roundhouse,
which he has since built. No one alive knew how to build such
a roundhouse.

8. Fusion with Elements of Nature

A graduate student dreamed he saw himself in a stone in Yosemite National Park. When he recognized his face there, the stone
dissolved and turned into several other animals. He woke up
laughing, exclaiming, "Everything is so beautiful." A few weeks
later he designed an ambitious graduate research project of trek-
king the hills of Nepal to determine the feasibility of using solar
cookers to replace the rapidly dwindling supplies of firewood.
Six months later he was in Nepal.

Visiting an old-growth redwood forest in northern California,
a woman reported being "drawn up into a tree." During the next
few moments she said she felt as though her body and the tree's
were one, and she understood what it was like to be a tree. She
has since become an outspoken advocate for saving old-growth
forests.

UNDERSTANDING
MANIFESTATIONS OF POWER

When a person who is in a compassionate and receptive state of
mind visits a special place and expresses respect for its power,
unusual things can happen, sometimes immediately, sometimes

later. If you believe that the earth itself is alive, you might say that such occurrences are an affirmation or reward given by nature in return for your expression of love.

Just what happens can vary widely, but the alchemical process of power being manifested is the same in each case. A symphony orchestra generates awesome power and energy when it plays in perfect accord, due to the number of harmonies struck among the instruments as well as to the composition itself. The same is true for the special magic between places and people. When ego boundaries relax, extraordinary harmonies between the inner self and the outer world become possible, resulting in lightning bolts of energy between the person and the nature kingdom. Like musical notes, these harmonic pulses create ripples that permeate all of life's many planes, causing numinous events to occur and new personal understandings to be made. Jungian analyst Marie-Louise von Franz has commented:

"It is being more and more firmly established that parapsychological phenomenona occur mainly in the surroundings of an individual whom the unconscious wants to take a step in the development of consciousness."[13]

In this respect, you might say that sacred places are amplifiers of being that make the experiences of transformation more profound, vivid, and predictable.

We are co-creators in a vast, intertwined network of energies and information, seeking to becoming who we really are and then to express ourselves. Power ultimately results from our achieving greater self-awareness and self-expression. Our minds can extend far beyond our bodies, and we can, and do, change the world from the inside out. This view is not widely held in the West, because, according to Elmer and Alyce Green at the Menninger Foundation, who have probably done more research with people with exceptional abilities than anyone else in the world, we are used to a myopic view of how humans function.

The Greens remark, "The persons who are most aware of their own normally unconscious processes are the ones who seem to most easily control their own nervous systems and physiological processes (heart, blood flow, brainwaves, pain) and who also seem to have the greatest extrasensory awareness of others, and the greatest ability to generate OUTS events, that is, to demonstrate psychokinetic powers."[14]

People ask if they can get a "bad trip" from visiting a sacred place. Legend has it that if you spend a night on top of Mount Patrick Couglin in England, you come down the next morning as a poet or a madman. Lakotas say that only people like Crazy Horse or Sitting Bull would seek a vision on Harney Peak in the Black Hills of South Dakota, because the power of the place is so great. People who go up on a sacred mountain and try to do their own vision-quest ritual, fasting for four or five days without proper supervision and training, could get into trouble if they start to have experiences they're not prepared for. But a far more risky power-seeking experience is some of the new-age instant-power-and-enlightenment seminars, which frequently blow people's minds open without properly trained support or guidance from people who understand transpersonal realms. Power can be sought, but it should not be taken lightly.

The only person I've met who has gone to a sacred place and come away feeling depressed was a woman who went to the Great Pyramid. She told me she felt deeply depressed for six months afterward. A pyramid is an archetypal symbol of power. Questioning her, I found that while visiting the Pyramid she had become aware of how powerless she had felt most of her life. After her depression began to lift, she began to take classes in assertiveness training and felt better about herself than ever.

A visit to a sacred place is a little like walking into a Rorschach ink-blot test: What you find is truth. The Sufis of the Middle East say that if a good person undertakes a pilgrimage, it will always make him better. If a bad person undertakes a pilgrimage, it may make him better or worse.

EMPOWERMENT OF PLACE

If you go to a special place and have a transcendent experience, what does it do for you? The first value is that it forever changes your view of yourself, the universe, and nature. Following a spiritual experience at a special place all of nature becomes forever after a "cosmic sacrality," said Mircea Eliade.

The second value is that it enables you to catch glimpses of possibilities in the future, as well as better understand the past and present. All planners, architects, and landscape architects should be required to spend time at sacred places. Artists of all persuasions flock to them in hopes of being inspired, even blessed.

The third value is that you discover special alignments of power that forever continue in your life with connections back to those magical experiences. An animal, plant, or stone that comes to you during a time of solitude at a sacred place is a revelation of kinship with nature that adds energy and power to your life.

A fourth value is that during moments of magic in nature you may be blessed by receiving guidance or creative inspiration. Visiting the Iglulik Eskimos in the 1920s, Danish explorer Knud Rasmussen was told by an old Eskimo shaman named Najagnea: "The best magic words are those which come to one when one is alone out among the mountains. These are always the most powerful in their effects. The power of solitude is great beyond understanding."[15]

Perhaps the wisest advice on seeking power words from sacred places comes from the venerable sage Winnie the Pooh, who counsels in *The House at Pooh Corner,* "Poetry and hums aren't things which you get, they're things that get you. And all you can do is to go where they can find you."

When I was in American Samoa, I spent some time with a *tautai,* a master fisherman, who was living proof of the power of man and nature working in harmony. As he sat on a black volcanic stone protruding from a sparkling white beach with the teal-blue tepid tropical ocean lapping at his feet, he would often be singing a refrain. I asked him what he was singing. "A fish song," he replied. Later I learned that this special song had come when he was making an offering to a special sacred place that is said to be the home of spirits of the ocean.

There is a saying in Samoa that "the fish do the will of the chief fisherman," and to achieve this level of proficiency as a fisherman, "you have to learn to think like a fish," the man told me with a warm smile. For him, each puff of wind, passing seabird, and cloud formation was a message from the spirits. His handwoven basket traps were spells of enchantment. When he lifted his traps and they were filled with bright-red, big-eyed reef fish, I understood what he was saying.

SUGGESTION: Choose one species of animal you feel represents qualities of personal power you would like to embody. Study the animal. What does it eat? What kinds of habitats does it frequent? What behaviors does it engage in? What sounds does it make? Set aside an hour or two and imagine you are one of this species. Eat as it would. Visit the places it frequents. See if you can mimic its calls. When native people want to develop skills to track a certain animal, they often advise that you learn to walk in its tracks first. When you do this, you gain insights into how this animal uses its special gifts to make the best use of the habitat available, which is an expression of personal power. How could you be a little more like an eagle, a rabbit, a deer, or a bear in your life and feel more empowered? Some people who do this exercise make masks of their animals, put on music, and dance as if they were the animal. If you do this, the Easter bunny and Halloween costumes will never be the same to you again.

TAPPING INTO THE POWER OF PLACE

The *I Ching* counsels us about the power of place: "Heaven and earth determine the places. The holy sages fulfill the possibilities of the places. Through the thoughts of men and the thoughts of spirits, people are enabled to participate in these possibilities."

Some of the people who are best at working with the powers of special places are shamans. Power in the Native American world has names such as *Wakan, Orenda, Kupuri, Manitou,* and *Pokunt.* These translate as a fusion of spiritual and material consciousness that manifests energies to make things happen that are in accord with the highest purposes of life.

Rolling Thunder is someone who manifests powers as a result of nature kinship. In 1981, just prior to Rolling Thunder's first public lecture in the Pacific Northwest, two people came to me with an Indian boy who was hardly able to work. They explained that he had a lung infection and they pleaded with me to ask Rolling Thunder if he would do something. Earlier, Rolling Thunder had given me instructions that no healings would be done, but somehow I felt he should know about this request. I went backstage into a small room filled with the pungent smoke of burning sage, sweetgrass, and his corncob pipe. I told him about the boy, and he gazed up into the smoke, squinting his eyes in a peculiar way. Then he said matter-of-factly, "Tell him I won't promise anything, but have him sit in the first couple of rows."

There was a sellout crowd of eight hundred packed into Unity Church that night. The program began with a round of drumming and singing with four seated drummers and four of us standing, joining them in chants. Rolling Thunder said a prayer, addressing each of the directions and their powers.

He talked for a while, and then we drummed and sang. Then he talked awhile longer, and again we sang. With each round you could feel the energies building and building. Finally they seemed to reach a crescendo, and he told the drummers to start up again. Rolling Thunder pulled his eagle-feather wand out of his badger-skin medicine bag and began making passes through the air.

He spotted the ailing boy in the second row and he reached back over the top of the throbbing drum with his wand and made a scooping motion, as if gathering energy from the drum. He then thrust his wand, like a sword, toward the boy, who immediately began to cough. He repeated this gesture three more times, shooting thunderbolts of energy. Each time the boy coughed more.

The young Indian boy was now having a coughing fit, and he had to be carried to a back room. The thought crossed my mind of newspaper headlines the next morning reading, MEDICINE MAN KILLS BOY IN CEREMONY. A physician was present. They asked me for a box of tissues. I got one and then had to go back to the hall.

When I came back half an hour later, I found two large paper bags filled with tissues and paper towels that had been used for the boy to cough up phlegm into. He was a little shaky, but he got to his feet and left the room walking without any help, a beaming smile on his face.

A few months later I produced a lecture for Rev. Olga Worrall, an awesome spiritual healer. After the lecture a man with cancer came forward. She took his hand and said a few words of prayer. The next day he excitedly called to report that his tumor was gone! His only complaint was that during the night he had been so filled with energy that he could not sleep.

In the case of both Rolling Thunder and Olga Worrall, they spoke of how they had gained power through a lifelong series of special experiences that often involved visiting special places or having dreams about aspects of nature. In Rolling Thunder's tradition shamans seek special power songs and chants by praying for them at sacred places. In the Russian Orthodox church, where Olga Worrall was raised, spiritual power is invoked through use of the icons displayed on the walls of the church. As

Olga showed me one day in a beautiful old church in Seattle, the icons of the Russian church include shocks of wheat, pictures of trees, and animals, as well as Christian figures.

The idea that the greatest power comes from ego control clearly does not explain the work of truly powerful people. In his best-selling book *Megatrends,* John Naisbitt says, "Whenever a new technology is introduced into society, there must be a counterbalancing human response," otherwise we go out of balance and lose harmony with nature. At the other end of the balance scale for modern technology is the reclamation of shamanism, which represents mankind's mastery of nature kinship. This does not mean giving up modern religions, but rather doing as the Russian Orthodox church does: blending together nature religions with others to create a powerful syncretism that rekindles the ability of people to know firsthand direct contact with the spirit.

Spiritual healing is one of a number of unusual powers that shamans may possess. One of the most well known and controversial aspects of shamanic powers is the ability to influence the weather.

The Greek philosopher Plutarch observed that unusually heavy rains seemed to fall after major battles. The hypothesis of that day was that this was the work of the gods, who wished to purify the battlefield of gore and blood.

Weather modification is a dangerous business. A single thunderstorm can dump 125 million gallons of water. There is enough electrical energy in the average thunderstorm to meet the power needs of the United States for twenty minutes, the equivalent of a 120-kiloton nuclear bomb. The average lightning bolt Thor hurls down has 30 amperes of electricity, and the resulting heat is in excess of 54,000 degrees Fahrenheit. It seems hard to believe that human thought can influence the weather, and yet there are so many examples of apparent successes in weather-working by shamans that it is hard to dismiss this possibility.

When President Gerald Ford was supposed to spend his

Christmas vacation at Vail, Colorado, in 1976, and there wasn't enough snowfall for skiing, Thetis Cloud, a member of the Sundance People of the Southern Ute tribe, agreed to perform a snow-making ceremony. Cloud performed the ceremony on December 20. Following the ritual no blizzard dropped two to three feet of snow within three days, as tradition said should happen, but to the delight of President Ford and other skiers, two feet of new snow fell within the next two weeks.

The snow-making ceremony was requested by Bob Parker, senior vice president of Vail Associates, based on previous success with snow-making ceremonies. The last time the Sundance People had been called to Vail to help get the ski season under way was in 1963, when Minnie Cloud, the elder of the Cloud Clan, led a ceremony that was promptly followed by two feet of snow, Vail Associates reported.[16]

In 1989 Copper Mountain ski resort in Colorado called upon the services of Muskogee Indian medicine man Marcellus Bear Heart Williams to pray for snow to make Thanksgiving skiing possible. Bear Heart chanted, drummed, smoked his pipe, and prayed. Soon it began to snow, and the skiing season began on schedule. The delighted resort owners then admitted that on two previous occasions they had retained Bear Heart to keep unwanted rain away from their slopes, and no rain had fallen.[17]

Weather-working is an ancient art, a manifestation of extraordinary powers, or *siddhi* in Sanskrit. The sages of India have long known of exceptional abilities but advise they are not to be taken lightly or developed too quickly. A person can force things to happen, they say, but the greatest power is a manifestation of unity with the highest purposes of life, which one must first learn. Sages don't always pray for rain, they pray for unity with God's will. *Moksha*, or wisdom, comes before *siddhi*, they teach, otherwise power can be misused.

In the final analysis the greatest personal power seems to arise not so much from gaining absolute control over people and situations but from cultivating the ability to channel and focus natural energies over which a person has only partial control. The tool that accomplishes this end for individuals and groups most effectively is ritual.

Exorcising Evil
from a Sacred Mountain

In perhaps the most important modern study of evil in recent times, Erich Fromm's *The Anatomy of Human Destructiveness,* the wise psychologist concluded that "destructiveness and cruelty are not instinctual drives . . . but passions rooted in the total existence of man," primarily fueled by fear and hatred.

Perhaps the most frightening evil person of all is someone whose style of evil blends with the spirit of a sacred place. My neighbor, Mount Tamalpais in Marin County just north of San Francisco, is an ancestral Miwok Indian sacred mountain. Tamalpa, the reclining maiden, awaits her suitor, Mount Diablo to the east, to come join her. On its western flank lie the giant redwoods of Muir Woods National Monument. Its 2,571-foot summit is the highest elevation in the Bay Area. The power of this mountain seems to move people to want to perform rituals there.

In the fall of 1980 seven women runners and hikers were brutally murdered on the slopes of Mount Tam. They were forced off hiking trails at gunpoint, forced to disrobe and kneel down, and then were shot or stabbed to death and raped by a killer, who performed ceremonies as part of his gruesome murders. Places of power, I believe, are like archetypes of consciousness that can be used for good or for evil ends. This killer seemed to embody the shadow of the mountain's power.

"A psychopathic killer is loose," declared the Marin County sheriff at a press conference. A wave of terror swept through the community. At the home of Anna and Lawrence Halprin on the north slope of Mount Tamalpais, a group of people assembled, wondering what they could do as their neighbors purchased locks and guns in record numbers. Internationally acclaimed for her pioneering innovations in dance, Anna Halprin stood up and said, "We have to do something to reclaim the mountain, something like an exorcism."

At the time Anna and Lawrence, an equally famous landscape architect, were conducting a series of community classes entitled "A Search for Living Myths Through Dance and Environment." They asked their students if they would help create a ritual for the most powerful source of myth around, the mountain, to free the shroud of terror that veiled its slopes like the coastal fog that billows in off Grandmother Ocean to the west.

On April 10, 1981, Anna Halprin's Tamalpa Institute produced a spellbinding dance performance, "In the Mountain: On the Mountain." Costumed dancers portraying the winds, water, earth, and fire whirled about the room, embodying the forces of nature and calling on their powers to join with those assembled. Seven women dressed in flowing white robes solemnly passed across the stage, depicting the victims of the "Trailside Killer." Anna herself, at age sixty, danced the lead role, playing both the killer and one of the victims before a rapt audience.

Charged with the energy of the dance, the next day Lawrence and Anna lead a group of eighty people to the top of Mount Tamalpais. A sheriff's car bearing a sketch of the killer on the driver's door greets them at the summit parking lot. Warnings are grimly posted on all the trails.

Lawrence instructs them to join hands and walk together as a human chain the quarter mile to the very top of the mountain. At the summit they stand in silence for a few moments, encircling it with their bodies. Several people offer prayers for peace and safety. Then they regroup in the parking lot.

The sheriff tells them, "Stay in small groups so that the killer can't sneak into your group and pick you off." Overhead a police helicopter buzzes by as the group began its descent down the mountain's fire trail.

Lawrence takes the lead, shouting out instructions over a

bullhorn. People are carrying bamboo staffs, playing musical instruments, and dancing. Many of the dancers from the previous night's performance wear their costumes from the night before. Anna carries a drum, moving through the group beating out a rhythm to keep people together. Suddenly one woman breaks into hysterical sobs, screaming the killer has infiltrated her group. A quick check proves this isn't so. Kush, a cantor from the previous night's ritual, begins to chant a refrain, "Life is sacred . . . hold fast our lands to your sacred ways." He keeps chanting and chanting loudly, moving through the group until everyone is chanting together. Calm is restored, and they move on.

Coming to a wide place in the trail, Anna and a group of five children do a spontaneous dance. A eucalyptus tree is produced and planted with a simple ceremony. Then the group moves on.

Six miles later they emerge from the woods into downtown Kentfield, ending the march where the dance had been held the night before. Everyone is safe. The sacred circle has been completed. The mountaintop and the valley below are united by a ritual act. The highest powers have been sought with sincerity.

A few days later an anonymous phone tip leads police to arrest a suspect. The killings stop. An uneasy sense of peace seems slowly to grow back onto the mountain.

Several months later Anna's Tamalpa Institute is visited by the one-hundred-year-old Huichol Indian shaman Don José Matsuwa from Mexico. Don José asks to be taken to the top of the mountain. Reaching the top of the mountain, the old man breaks into tears. He says that years ago he had a dream where he saw this very mountain. "This mountain is one of the most powerful places on earth," he declares. He takes an eagle feather from his medicine bag and delivers a blessing. Then he is silent for a minute, listening, watching, hoping for an answer. Finally he turns to the Halprins and says, "What you did was very important, but for it to be successful, you must return to this mountain every year for five years and perform a ceremony."

For the next four years Anna Halprin creates an annual dance ritual honoring Mount Tamalpais and the women killed on the mountain. Runners ascending the mountain in the ceremony say they feel like they are being "pulled up the mountain by a strange force." On the summit, while prayers and speeches are made, birds flock in the trees overhead and sing joyously. Something very special is happening.

As the fifth annual ceremony begins to take form, there's an eerie note of irony as the convicted Trailside Killer is about to be sentenced. His trial has been delayed because he had to be tried for other murders near Santa Cruz first.

On Easter Sunday morning one hundred runners ascend Mount Tamalpais on half a dozen trails. The first fifteen hundred feet of the mountain is covered by heavy fog, as if nature were reminding us of the heaviness that hung over the mountain five years before. Once we are above the fog, the sky is clear and the sun is shining down on the coastal fog, making it look like an aerial ocean. One group of runners dressed in white chant "Ho, ho, ho" all the way up the mountain and are led by Anna, who is carrying an eagle feather on a long staff. They are the cloud spirits as they emerge from the puffy white low-flying stratus clouds.

On the summit prayers are said by a Sufi, a rabbi, a Christian minister, and several Native Americans, including Lakota actor Floyd Westerman, who later played wise old Chief Ten Bears in the movie *Dances with Wolves.* "We must take this spirit back down the mountain," Anna says, holding back tears. Right on cue a raven swoops by, loudly calling out *owrk, owrk, owrk,* and everyone cheers.

For one week Anna trains one hundred people from all walks of life who will dance together in the final performance, "Circle the Earth." On Saturday evening they are joined by four hundred "witnesses," who will both watch and become part of the performance.

The witnesses meet outside the gym where the performance

will take place, and at 8:30 p.m. Anna leads them down a pathway of lighted candelabra to the gymnasium. Inside, brightly decorated banners hang from the ceiling everywhere. It is like walking into the Northern Lights. The bodies of the one hundred dancers are strewn everywhere, lying motionless on the floor. Anna has us weave through them, explaining that they are the spirits of the mountain waiting to come to life.

As the audience takes its seats, a man runs out with a bull roarer, a flat stick whirled on a string in a circle that makes sounds like peals of thunder. Slowly the dancers rise to their feet. The late Martha Graham once said that dance is most effective when dancers become gods. You can feel the gods' presence as the dance begins.

Slowly the dance builds, a choreographed piece that shows with physical movement the evolution of life on earth. The music comes to a crescendo as all the dancers merge together in the center of the floor and form the mountain with their bodies.

Now Anna, dressed in white, appears. The mountain dissolves, and she warns us that some powerful energies are about to be mobilized. "We will become killers and the killed to show how these parts are in all of us. It will not be pretty, but the way you come to master your own dark side is to face it."

This time as the music builds, before us one hundred people are killed and become killers. To protect the audience from the carnage, each person is given a white mask to wear. Then a single loud drumbeat sounds out, and everyone falls to the ground. We see what a nuclear bomb might do.

The dancers now form two lines, like a birth canal, and invite the audience to file down the channel and join them. At the other end Anna is dancing with a beautiful young girl of six or seven all dressed in white.

Then everyone forms a giant circle to re-create the run for peace, which has become a standard element of this ritual. At the culmination religious leaders from half a dozen faiths step forward and offer prayers. The evening culminates as everyone sings together:

> *May the peace that we love be what we feel.*
> *May the peace that we feel be what we do.*

The "Circle the Earth" dance ritual described here in its 1986 premiere performance has now become an international peace celebration, performed annually in at least forty countries around the world. Its power to move minds and bodies to action springs from a source beyond self, showing us how recovering our roots in myths, symbols, and sympathies with nature can lead mortals to accomplish the seemingly impossible. The potential to become more powerful resides in each of us, waiting to be developed, for as Frank Waters reminds us in his moving tale of Southwestern Indian life, *The Man Who Killed the Deer,* "Nothing is simple and alone. We are not separate and alone. The breathing mountains, the living stones, each blade of grass, the clouds, the rain, each star, the beasts, the birds and the invisible spirits of the air—we are all one, indivisible. Nothing that any of us does but affects us all."[18]

SUGGESTION: The previous exercises in this book have guided you to discover a whole series of symbols of nature that have special meaning for you. Refer back to the exercises you have done and what you've found to be your tree, place, plant, animal, and mineral symbols of nature. Try bringing them all together into one design that seems to express who you are in good relation to nature. You may want to include symbols from your ancestry as well, including those from your clan or family tree. One person became so inspired by this integration exercise that he went home and carved a personal totem pole.

Chapter Nine

KEEPING NATURE'S MAGIC
IN YOUR LIFE

*The ancestral wisdoms of the human race
taught us to look at the Earth as alive
and not an inanimate object of aggression and
pillage. For countless ages, harmony between
man and the biosphere was the basis of
human living. We are witnessing now the
effects of the loss of this delicate
balance . . . [we need] a new vision, a new loyalty,
an Earth patriotism as strong as any national patriotism to relieve
the distress of our ailing and exhausted planet.*

—U.N. SECRETARY-GENERAL JAVIER PEREZ DE CUELLAR
Keynote Speech, World Forum on Human Survival, Moscow, January 1990

Seeking inspiration to conclude this book, I retreat to Point Reyes National Seashore, about an hour's drive north of my home, with a small group of friends. There are a few patches of high clouds as we leave. By the time we get there, the sky is completely overcast, and a light, misty rain is falling.

As we park our cars at Limantour Beach, the rain begins to fall steadily. "Great!" we exclaim, strapping on packs. "This will keep the crowds away." We set off down the beach.

Soon we are passing flocks of jet-black scoters bobbing up and down in the breakers. Thoughts of the telephone, television, bills, and so forth begin to slip away as our caravan trudges through the sand. The wind is now gusting from the west, and the low coastal fog is mixing with the rain, sweeping us up in a gentle, salty mist that tastes like tears as droplets flow down our cheeks into our mouths. Along the way I gather kelp fronds, plantain leaves, and miner's lettuce to put into the evening stew. We take sips of well water to harmonize with the world below the ground. Arriving at our campsite, I take out a little cornmeal and toss it in the bushes, making a gesture of respect to the place and its powers, explaining that I am there to seek inspiration to finish my book. Almost immediately an osprey flies by clutching a big fish in its talons, obviously a good omen.

We pitch our tents at the Coast Camp walk-in site, and our spirits are slightly dampened now by the chilling fog and rain. Turning to technology to provide warmth and nourishment, we find that our first stove produces only a dim flicker. The second catches fire with a kerosene leak, nearly creating a tragedy. The third coughs and sputters and goes out. The firewood is all soaked. Suddenly the dream of a great potluck stew enjoyed beside a roaring campfire fades away in the cold, wet, windy night air.

Shivering with cold, my teenage son, Andrew, decides to retreat to the tent and crawl into his sleeping bag. We hover around the one tiny glowing flame of the only working camp stove, trying to heat everything from hands to hot dogs to coffee. A few minutes later Andrew lets out a yelp as if a bear is attacking him. There are no bears at Point Reyes, but we go to see what's up. Father had left the tent flap open. A skunk has crawled inside the tent and walked on top of Andrew. The message from the nature spirits is very clear: Back to civilization!

René Dubos observed in his later years,

I now realize how much my life would have been enriched by longer and more intimate contacts with wilderness. The experience of nature in a native prairie, a desert, a primeval forest, or high mountains not crowded with tourists is qualitatively different from what it is in a well-tended meadow, wheat field, an olive grove, or even in the high Alps. Humanized environments give us confidence because nature has been reduced to the human scale, but the wilderness in whatever form almost compels us to measure ourselves against the cosmos.[1]

In a century the United States has gone from a rural nation where more than 90 percent of the people lived in the country to the polar opposite—more than 90 percent of the people live in cities today. These urbanites may spend more than three quarters of life indoors. Considering the ever-growing power of modern technology and the fact that human creativity arises from our inner psyche, we must more than ever before keep ourselves firmly rooted in nature kinship to avert ecological apocalypse. And because of our numbers and living patterns, we must establish this harmony with nature while spending most of our time in an increasingly urbanized world.

I believe there are three great challenges for modern society to meet if we want to keep nature's magic alive in our lives at all times. The first is to remain in harmony with nature yet not forget that we are also rational humans; that is, we need to avoid what some call becoming lost in God. The second challenge is to live out our lives with the understanding that we are part of a wondrous system, linked to all other creatures by a network stretching far into other worlds, and that for every action there is a corresponding pulsation in the entire web of life. The third is to create a healthy, renewing, sustainable human community based on successfully achieving the first two goals.

The thrust of this book has been to describe an honest psychology of how one establishes and maintains an intimate link with nature so that nature serves as a source of knowledge and health throughout the journey of life. Many people find that accepting this paradigm and following the suggestions offered enriches their lives. But we cannot live in the wild places, at least not for long. Countless people know the letdown of coming home from a retreat to nature. Many others live lives of "quiet desperation," as Thoreau described modern life, surviving by escaping to wild places in every free moment. The real challenge of creating a sustainable society is to structure life so that the healing energies of nature can be brought right into the places where we live and work and be preserved by all the social institutions that are necessary to support vital human community. Accomplishing this goal calls for more than what we've been doing in the name of ecology as a social movement.

Toward a New Environmentalism

Bill Moyers, at the Social Movement Empowerment Project in San Francisco, has been studying social transformation for a number of years. He sees a predictable pattern in the emergence of new values.[2] First, conditions for change become clear, usually because existing institutions fail to address a problem adequately. This often begins with a dramatic event, such as the 1969 Santa Barbara oil spill or the 1989 Alaskan oil spill in Prince William Sound. As people become aware of a problem and start to share a need for change, they get organized, usually along political lines, and build to some kind of an early crescendo. An example of this is Earth Day 1970, when twenty million people participated in peaceful demonstrations all across the United States; *ecology* became a household word; the EPA was created; membership in environmental groups skyrocketed; and ecology laws were passed.

Next is a feeling of powerlessness. As the fires of hot controversy cool with time and as a result of only partial responses to the protest, public concern—and media coverage—moves on to other hot issues. Without a critical mass of people to pursue it, an issue soon disappears from view. Studies show that if 20 percent of the people of a group accept an idea, it's not likely to disappear. If the cause doesn't die after the initial peak of popularity, gradual systemic reorganization that ultimately reaches right down to the roots of society will occur, and the values embodied in the initial protest will become lasting, living ethics that become integrated into the entire culture.

Environmentalists have been around for a long, long time. In fact, ecological concern may be the oldest form of social activism. When modern science and religion came to the United States, we killed off most of the original truly committed environmentalists (or put them on reservations). Our first modern environmental activists were artists—writers such as John Muir, Henry David Thoreau, and John Burroughs; and painters such as John James Audubon and Mark Catesby. With their sensitivity they recognized what we were losing, and they described or portrayed natural beauty and the destruction of creatures and resources in ways that moved our emotions, triggering the formation of environmental organizations like the Sierra Club and the National Audubon Society. Teddy Roosevelt and Gifford Pinchot launched the conservation movement, which sought to preserve woods and wildlife and fight soil erosion. They introduced science into resource management and put us on the right track, although too late to save the passenger pigeon, the heath hen, the Carolina parakeet, the great pine forests of the Midwest, and (nearly) the buffalo.

The volcanic eruption of the modern environmental movement in 1970 came as a kind of fourth great wave of the collective unconscious, which reminded us that something was wrong with the American dream. Racial inequality, sexual discrimination, the Vietnam War—a triple whammy. After Earth Day 1970, science became political, thanks to Margaret Mead, Barry Commoner, Paul Ehrlich, David Brower, Gaylord Nelson, and Edmund Muskie. And environmental law emerged as a potent weapon to save the earth, thanks to Ralph Nader and Vic Yannaconne.

The 1970s and '80s were a time of deep soul-searching for many people, when the inner environment became more important than the external one. Experimenting with Eastern religions, drugs, and humanistic and transpersonal psychology, millions of people opened what Aldous Huxley called the doors of perception. We discovered that self-awareness was the key to taking control of our lives and that spirituality was something we could know firsthand. The environment slipped off into a backwater, surfacing only in Jacques Cousteau's television documentaries and the daring escapades of Greenpeace.

The seventies and eighties might well be called the decades of growing awareness. Millions discovered their inner lives, feelings, and emotions. The mass media became capable of linking the world in an instantaneous global communication network. And sophisticated environmental monitoring instruments such as the gas chromatograph were invented, allowing us to perceive and understand chemical pollution and global climatic changes no senses could detect. Suddenly we became aware that we were destroying nature and ourselves. In response, organic and health foods became very popular, and a massive health and fitness industry mushroomed.

Chernobyl and the Alaskan oil spill rekindled old fires long dormant. Earth Day 1990 attracted more than two hundred million people in 140 countries. Memberships in environmental organizations again swelled, and people everywhere began talking about the rain forests, acid rain, and global warming. But there was also a backlash.

"Earth Day 1990 was a media event," cried the protesters who chained themselves to the Golden Gate Bridge the day after Earth Day 1990 in San Francisco had brought over 100,000 people to a rock concert at Crissey Field. On the other coast a violent anti–Wall Street protest took place in the heart of New York's financial district, charging environmental groups with selling out to big business. When the shadow comes out, there's always a grain of truth. But the real issue the protest raised was how terrified people feel about the future. When people feel powerless, terror and terrorism surface most often.

But Earth Day 1990 wasn't an angry political protest as it was in 1970. The second generation came together to show with their feet that they cared. Emerging after two decades of feeling power-less, they wanted music and entertainment to boost their spirits so that they could begin to make a personal effort—such as recycling household garbage—and feel that it made a difference.

Rallies need causes and, better yet, fresh enemies to focus on. Aside from Exxon, good clear-cut enemies were hard to find in 1990. Today's toxic pollution is not nearly as dramatic as the detergent-laden wastewaters that flowed into Lake Erie in the 1960s, the flames that licked across the Cuyahoga River in 1969, or the huge dustfalls of particulate matter that once filled the air over most big cities. Instead we're now dealing more with over-flowing garbage dumps (here and in countries abroad that take our garbage), the destruction of the rain forests and their indige-nous species, the pollution of the oceans, global climatic change, and toxins not perceived by the five senses. In many cases scien-tists, television, and computers are essential to let us know that something's wrong at all. When it's not clear who and where the enemy is, anger turns into fear, terror, cynicism, and confusion.

Think globally and act locally is the rallying cry of our times. When each person recycles, conserves energy, buys organic pro-duce, reuses paper bags, and other simple things that help the environment, collectively it makes a difference. People want to help out, which is why the save-the-earth books with their simple suggestions sold so well around Earth Day 1991. But there is no immediate guarantee that our individual actions will collectively succeed, and the media tend to focus on disasters more than on success stories. Maintaining our Earth Day good behavior won't result from simply overloading people with information and education. What modern people lack is not information but an intensity of feeling for it and the knowledge that their lives are worthwhile.

Concerts are fun, but they tend to be like one-night stands, fading quickly with no follow-through. The existing environmen-tal organizations working on political action—mounting legal challenges to pollution, preserving rare species and beautiful

natural areas, and churning out documentary movies and magazines—are important to ecological conservation, but to develop
a sustainable society that lives and creates in harmony with
nature, we need some much broader-based environmental-action
strategies to form a working ecological ethic which prevails every
day of the year.

There is a tendency to want to create ethics by preaching
them. Selling self-righteous *shoulds* is always a risky business.
The results of such strategies are generally short-lived and heavily
dependent upon charismatic leadership, terrorism, or law en-
forcement to make them work at all. All too often we discover
later that those who preach ethics don't practice them.

Building a viable ethic of nature kinship that produces long-
term ecological sustainability will depend on at least four conditions being met:

1. Each person must know in his or her bones that the ethical
   behaviors are appropriate. It must be an internally accepted
   code not based on any external authority figures to keep it
   alive. Awe, not guilt, is the psychological incentive of successful ethical codes in the long run.
2. The ethic must be supported by the collective interaction of
   mutually supportive elements spread throughout the entire
   cultural system—a web of agreements communicated in
   many forms, both linear and nonlinear, that all serve as a
   constant reminder that the ethic must be central to thought
   and action for survival.
3. Cultural ethics that work in the long run arise from mythic
   sentiments woven into mutually supportive networks of social
   agreements and ideals, which are periodically renewed. In the
   long run myths and symbols, more than words, shape our
   reality, and rites are more important than rallies for reliably
   shaping human actions.
4. Those who embrace the sentiments of the new ecological ethic
   should not be at a disadvantage compared with those who do

not hold them. The smart businesses of tomorrow will be those that both make a profit and are examples of ecological integrity. Self-sacrifice in the name of social responsibility all too often means self-castration and decreased power for those people who assert they hold environmental values dearly.

Throughout the pages of this book I've described a psychology of nature kinship, described its value, and offered suggestions about how to increase your kinship ties with nature. Many of the suggestions involve personal exercises for discovering identity, meaning, purpose, and power; accessing healing energies; and tapping into the significance of place. The purpose of entering into the state of mind where nature is a teacher and healer is to guide you to act in accord with nature, whatever you may do for a living—whether you are a teacher, businessperson, architect, entertainer, or homemaker.

Maximizing nature kinship calls for engaging in acts that are ultimately rituals—sequences of communicative acts designed to create certain results. To be human is to ritualize, regardless of what you call it. Rituals can take on all kinds of human forms, and every architectural design, city plan, and landscape development is a ritual too. Even though we are now in the modern information age, we cannot escape the human need to ritualize. In fact, more than ever, we need to build a whole system of mutually supportive ritual actions to weave a dynamic spell of human-nature kinship that brings beauty and magic into every act we make.

Regaining Our Roots in Ritual

Every year since 1900 the people of American Samoa have held an enormous Flag Day celebration on April 17 to commemorate their becoming a Trust Territory of the United States. When Margaret Mead wrote *Coming of Age in Samoa* in the late 1920s, about 5,000 people lived on these seven tiny tropical islands. In

1984, when I was in American Samoa, more than 8,000 people participated in the Flag Day ceremonies at the football field in Pago Pago, another 4,000 watched in person, and most of the rest of the 33,000 present-day population watched via live television. The sense of community was awesome!

Reminiscent of Band Day at the University of Michigan football stadium, when the playing field is filled with high school marching bands at halftime, the people of Samoa come to Flag Day in large marching groups with all the members of each group wearing the same color lava-lava skirts, each singing a particular song that represents the group's spirit. Each village has its own songs and dances, and so do the women who work at the tuna canneries, the various schools, the police force, most church parishes, and each of the *aigas,* or extended families, represented in the celebration.

As I stood there in this sea of rainbow-colored singing and dancing bodies lifting their voices in praise of the beauty of Samoa and its people, I came to understand for the first time just how right Joseph Campbell was when he said, "It is possible that the failure of mythology and ritual to function effectively in our civilization may account for the high incidence among us of the malaise that has led to the characterization of our times as 'the age of anxiety.' "[3]

The advent of each new season, the arrival of migrating fish and game, the cycles of the sun and the moon, the sowing of seed in the spring and the harvesting of crops in the fall, and all the major stages of the life cycle—all were once marked with a pageantry of songs, symbols, dances, and ritual acts woven together in a tapestry of awe and magic that reinforced cultural norms, eased the flow of life, and harmonized people with nature. The ongoing procession of rituals acted like glue to bind people together with common values. They served as an amplifier to facilitate entering altered states of consciousness. And they were a way to vent human emotions and to channel these sentiments into cultural wisdom. Originally rituals were both celebrations and an excellent way of preserving community mental health. Looking at sustainable societies throughout history and around the world, it is evident that one of the most integral elements of their makeup is the heavy use of ceremony and ritual to keep their cultures renewed and in harmony with nature.

As societies become industrialized, the old gods of magic, mystery, and ecstasy that kept the myths alive are replaced by a new pantheon. The drum becomes a clock. Church and state separate. Priests of the churches mechanically replicate ritual acts that seldom afford congregations the chance to transcend themselves or to discover personal meaning. Alcoholism and drug abuse increase to give people a new, easy, but unintegrated way of altering consciousness. Political officials cut ribbons, break champagne against new ships, and dig foundations with silver spades, and scientists perform standardized procedures to find the "truth," but their original roles—as priests and alchemists—have disappeared. Schedules take over as the ordering factor in daily life. The old unity in life fades away, to be replaced by predictable mechanization and fragmentation. Community spirit dwindles as dog-eat-dog competition takes over as the ethic of the day. Loneliness becomes more common, even though more of us live closer and closer together, and people harmonize with machines, instead of with natural cycles and patterns.

It's no coincidence that scholars began to cry out, "God is dead," as the age of machines blossomed. God never died, but our sense of the divine did as we harmonized with cogwheels instead of with the seasons, one's dreams, the rain, the sunrise, and the call of wild geese riding on the north wind.

The most effective rituals are those that are right for the times, the place, and the people. To regain our nature kinship, we need to invent new, more meaningful ritual forms on all levels to reconnect us with nature at every stage of the life cycle and in every season of the year. Looking around the world and historically, you can find examples that may serve to inspire you to create your own ceremonies or add to existing ones to ensure that nature isn't forgotten.

NATURE AND RITES OF PASSAGE

Among the Big Mountain Dineh (Navajo), when a child is born, it is taken outside and presented to the sun or moon. Then the afterbirth is hung in a special tree. Farther north in the Pacific Northwest, the Lummi tribe bathes newborns in the Grandmother Ocean, introducing them to their ancestral mother within hours of birth. Growing up among the Asmat Ou of Southeast Asia, children learn through stories, songs, dances, and rituals that they are one with the trees. A good adult is a "tree person." Cutting a tree requires a long ritual process, including planting several new ones to take its place. As you might expect, deforestation is unknown among the Asmat Ou.

As preparation for a life of ceremony and ritual among many Pueblo tribes, young children spend as much as nine months sitting in silence in an underground cave called a kiva. During this time they may be taught from time to time by an elder, but more important, in the silence they learn to listen. What they hear is the voice and heartbeat of their second mother, the earth. This education in interspecies communication with the earth has been beautifully described by Frank Waters in his memorable book *The Man Who Killed the Deer.*

In many cultures initiation into adulthood involves conquering fears of nature and turning the experience of being alone, possibly in dangerous wild places, into a search for self. A second proof of adulthood for men often involves the first kill of a large animal, such as a deer or a buffalo. One of the traditional requirements for women to be initiated as hula dancers in Hawaii was to meditate for a long time on palm trees swaying in the tropical breezes. Among many Indian tribes, women become initiated into adulthood through rituals linking them with fertile plants such as corn.

A marriage ceremony is a celebration of community in most cultures, but the honeymoon is frequently spent in seclusion in nature. This not only gives the couple privacy but also helps establish the link between love, sexuality, and beautiful natural places. In a modern age, honeymooning at Niagara Falls could symbolize taking the big step and letting go, with the presence of falling water suggesting loosening emotions.

Secret societies for men and women almost always have initiation experiences associated with nature. In many tribes, such as the Australian aborigines, people receive new names associated with nature as a result of successfully performing ordeals of initiation into secret orders. Modern versions of these old orders include the Masons, Elks, Eagles, and Moose clubs.

In death we return to nature as a body or ashes, returning to our origins. In traditional societies the place of burial is sacred. In American Samoa the graves of the highest chiefs are marked by large stone cairns on high hills overlooking quiet lagoons. And many American Indians believe that souls of the newborn and the deceased enter and exit the earth plane through special sacred places. Point Conception near Santa Barbara, California, is the Western Gate, and Assateague Island in Virginia is the Eastern Gate for many Native American Indians.

These brief sketches of ceremonial links to nature illustrate how nature kinship can be included at every stage of the life cycle, adding considerable depth in meaning and feeling as well as contributing to creating an overall land ethic. In addition to ceremonies to mark the stages of the life cycle, stories, games, music, and dance become blended into a tapestry of sentiments that move people to do the little things that collectively save the earth. And then as each season changes, we bring the community together to honor nature's ongoing procession, releasing old energies and inviting in new ones.

Origins of the Four Major
European Seasonal Celebrations

In most cultures large public events mark the passing of one season to another during the annual solar cycle. People in ancient times felt that during the solstices and equinoxes, cracks in the space-time frame open and allow easier contact between this world and the spirit world. Such events not only encouraged the expression of emotions and feelings associated with the changing moods of nature, releasing old energies to allow new ones to enter, but they also organized human behavior to capitalize on the availability of seasonal resources and stimulated creative expression. Further, they perpetuated mythic themes that in turn influenced cultural values and allowed spirituality to merge with material life in a practical and predictable manner.

A brief sketch of the four major seasonal celebrations follows, along with some insights into how they have changed over time. The timing of these rites varies from country to country, of course, and does not directly coincide with the the exact dates of the solstices and equinoxes in all cases. Use this background information as inspiration to create your own seasonal forms that weave the many elements of your community into a joyous celebration of communality and perpetuate harmony with nature.

EASTER

The sun "dances for joy" on Easter morning, if the devil doesn't get in the way—this is an old European belief about the magic of spring's appearance. While today people associate Easter with Christ's resurrection, a custom not established until the Middle Ages, Easter originally comes from the festival honoring the Saxon goddess Eostre, a northern form of the goddess Astarte, a nature deity whose origins date back to the Neolithic age. This holiday is also associated with the "Four Fires" of the year of

Celtic countries, which are traced to the Druids. The spring fire, Beltane, April 31, traditionally was held on May 1 and was named for the Norwegian god Bel or Baal, the son of Odin. In early times in northern Europe people lit bonfires on the tops of hills during each of the Four Fires to keep evil spirits at a distance when the veils between the worlds were thinner. Jumping over a fire supposedly cleansed away evil witchcraft. Today's Easter bunny has roots tracing back to the "moon hare," a familiar of the fertility goddess. An insight into the meanings of the Easter Bunny and colored eggs is seen in the traditional Czechoslovakian Easter custom of boys chasing girls with birch switches. When caught, to avoid a beating, the girls give the boys colored Easter eggs. It takes no imagination to guess what this symbolizes! In England the herb tansy was once used to flavor Easter cakes, its bitter taste associated with the ancient Hebrew religious foods of Passover. Lamb, a favorite food in many Easter meals and a symbol seen on a lot of Easter presents, is also an ancient pagan fertility symbol. The Hebrews sacrificed lambs at Easter time to honor the earth god.

SUMMER SOLSTICE

Solar observatories such as Stonehenge and the Rollwright circle have special markings to record the apex of the sun in the sky and the longest day of the year. While the summer season is beginning, with its warmth and abundance, many traditional peoples recognize death, for the summer solstice marks the beginning of the decline in hours of sunlight. For many people the celebrations held on that date are prayers to keep the sun's energy alive as long as possible.

The Druidic fire of the summer is Lugnasad, held around August 1. Its principal ceremonial form was a fiery wheel in a grove that people jumped over during periods of dancing.

For most people in the United States, the Fourth of July has really taken over as a summer solstice celebration, the fireworks in the sky symbolizing the bursts of artillery associated with our successful battles in the War of Independence. It's a time of community, family, and food that recognizes freedom and liberty. It's unfortunate that more efforts aren't made to weave back in some of the elements of nature that were once celebrated in the second of the Four Fires of the year.

FALL EQUINOX

Harvest festivals are common around the September 22 date of the fall equinox, but the traditional ceremony in Europe is All Hallows' Eve or Halloween, which comes over a month later on October 31. Halloween was originally a festival of the dead, when bright bonfires burned on hilltops to keep the powers of darkness at bay. Interestingly, the date for celebrating Halloween was moved from May 13 to October in the seventh century, as part of a Christianization of an earlier pagan celebration called Samhain, held on November 1. Samhain, the third great fire festival, marked the time when cattle were brought in from the pastures, and Samana—the Leveler, the Lord of Death, or the Grim Reaper—led the souls of the dead and a motley crew of ghosts, fairies, demons, hobgoblins, and witches to visit the living. The jack-o'-lanterns now so popular symbolize the will-o'-the-wisps out on All Hallows' Eve. The Grateful Dead rock band derives its name from this mythic theme. The custom of children going trick-or-treating combines two traditions. All Hallows' Eve celebrations were times of license, and people gave gifts to the poor who would otherwise destroy property when social standards were relaxed. Also, ancient traditions suggest that putting food out on Halloween night for the ghosts and other spirits will improve your chances of receiving the blessings and guidance of the spirits of the dead in your daily life.

CHRISTMAS

It was not until the fourth century that December 25 was declared the date of the birth of Christ. The earlier roots of the holiday that today has become so popular include the Norse Yule feast and the Roman Saturnalian orgy. The Druidic counterpart to Christmas is Imbolc, held on February 1. Its theme is to wash the face of the earth and prepare for the coming spring season, when the earth will again come into flower. The Christmas tree's origins trace back to shamanic times: The tree is universally considered the axis along which shamans travel between the three worlds in search of wisdom and power. The Yule log is a way of bringing the magic of the fourth great fire indoors to pray for warmth during the long dark winter. Mistletoe is an herb associated with many magical powers, including fertility. Its presence provides license to kiss freely, suggesting that Christmas was once a time of orgiastic festivities to help drive away the winter blues. Santa Claus became Saint Nicholas as part of the Christian church's political effort to take over the pagan rites. A bearded wise man in a red suit with a pointed hat who rides around in a magical sleigh driven by eight horned reindeer delivering blessings to people who behave righteously is a powerful statement about a shamanic process with roots far older than Christianity. It describes the magical spirit flight of the shaman, which enables the shaman to influence the course of human life through journeys to the otherworld, where he can take on spiritual power and be in many places at the same time. Some people feel the first Christmas trees were ritual sacrifices taken from the sacred groves of the Goddess.

A southern root of Christmas traces back to Rome and the Saturnalian orgies, when Saturn briefly became king and the poor received gifts from the rich. Role reversals were a common part of Saturnalian rites, which later became the Feast of Fools of the United Kingdom, a time when, in Scotland, the Lord of Misrule presided over a period of license and revelry.

Scandinavians celebrate the Santa Lucia festival in the days before winter solstice. At the head of the procession is a young teenage girl dressed in white with a tiara of white candles. She is followed by younger children dressed in white wearing pointed hats like those of witches and wizards, who are supposed to travel through the community bringing gifts of food. Here again Christianity changed things. Santa Lucia was originally a patron saint of Portuguese fishermen. I would suspect that the original festival had more to do with the lady of the lake or the mother of the animals coming with all her dwarves, elves, and trolls to bring cheer at the darkest time of the year in whatever fashion the needs of the people dictated.

Today these four great seasonal celebrations are all diminished by commercialism, loss of touch with their original spirit, and the conflict between their origins and modern Christianity's efforts to cut off our spiritual ties with nature. In South America new religions such as Santeria, modern voodoo, Umabanda, and others assert that all saints should have an equal place at the spiritual table. As the Christian church looks for ways to become more ecological, it will find itself reversing centuries of discrimination and practicing side by side with shamans, wizards, witches, pagans, and their images and idols. Christ, the Virgin Mary, and the Holy Ghost can and do get along very nicely with trees, jaguars, sheaves of wheat, stones, and flowing wells.

Seasonal celebrations are also often linked with special places in addition to conventional church buildings. Many traditional cultures included pilgrimages to springs, mountains, or caves as part of the overall process of honoring the passing seasons. In the United States we are seriously handicapped in establishing sacred places in natural settings to supplement regular services, since so much of the Indian religion and earth wisdom associated with it has been destroyed. In 1987 the Greater Church Council of Seattle issued a "letter of apology" to Indians, Eskimos, and

Aleuts of the Pacific Northwest for past harm done to traditional cultures and their religions by the Christian faith. This gesture was followed up by the bishops giving elk skins to medicine people to use for making drums for sweat-lodge ceremonies held in state prisons, and invitations to Indian spiritual leaders to join in ceremonies held at Christian churches. One outcome of this reconciliation process has been that Christian clergy and their congregations are now helping Indians to save endangered sacred Indian sites. It seems very appropriate that churches across the United States could reach out to Indian tribes and assist them with heritage preservation by joining with them to acknowledge certain places in nature as sacred places, perhaps even forming teams to help prevent vandalism there.

CREATING COMMUNITY

Community is the magical synergy of linking people in a common geographic area to accomplish things that one person could not accomplish alone. Community is created usually as a result of: 1) natural disasters; 2) confrontations with enemies; and 3) common shared values and norms that are catalyzed into action by shared sentiments and beliefs.

Before the days of modern communication and transportation technologies, people came together out of necessity to husk corn, build barns, and harvest crops, because otherwise they would not have survived. One of the best definitions of the attitude of how good, positive community spirit is cultivated is suggested by my friend Chung-Liang Al Huang, who likes to quote an ancient Chinese fable that says,

> Heaven and hell are exactly alike, in that each is an enormous banquet with every wonderful dish imaginable crowding the great round table. The diners are provided with chopsticks— five feet long!

In hell the diners give up struggling to feed themselves with these impossible tools and sit in ravenous frustration.

In heaven, everyone feeds the person across the table.[4]

Rituals used in service to communities at large where no one religious group predominates tend to be presented as festivals and carnivals. A review of these events around the United States and Canada shows that thousands of festivals of all kinds take place every year, as well as exposition shows, rodeos, sportsmen's shows, boat shows, art-and-craft expositions, dog shows, some conferences and symposia, and celebrations for the major seasons of the year. Each festival is an opportunity to establish and renew values of ecological stewardship.

Throughout the many Pueblo tribes of the Southwest there are cycles of seasonal celebrations where people and spirits fuse to energize the community, create a focus for tasks that need to be done, vent energies that build up when people live together in close quarters, and honor the spirits of nature and their mythic identities. At the Santa Clara pueblo, a home of the Tewa tribe, the word *gia* means "mother," a person who gives love, food, life, and health. *Gia,* however, has other connotations. *Gia* also means "the earth," "supernatural and religious symbols," "community, religious, social, and political leaders," "core family people," and "a person's biological mother."[5] These multiple meanings acknowledge that some people are gifted with a special medicine of helping people keep in harmony with nature, a social role that has been neglected in modern times, and they help underscore the importance of spirituality in arriving at an ecological conscience. Modern communities might benefit greatly from having a person who serves in a role like the community *gia.*

In American Samoa, a counterpart to the *gias* are the watchers of the springs and catchment basins that the village water supply comes from. In the old days women would take turns sitting beside the catchment basins and pools, guarding them from pigs, dogs, and other animals and periodically tossing hibiscus flowers on the surface to make the spirits of the springs happy. For sacred places, parks, recreation areas, historic sites, and all places of natural wonder, we could easily establish citizen watcher groups to protect natural beauty and give more people an active role in supporting the environment. Senior citizens, scouts, garden-club members, or other volunteers sweeping leaves or picking up trash would bring us closer to nature and a sense of community than a groundskeeper periodically coming by with an obnoxious gasoline-powered leaf blower.

Rituals are structured patterns of action designed to create certain results. Religions use rituals, but not all rituals have to be tied to a religious system. For example, athletes and performers of all persuasions commonly use rituals to get into the state of mind where personal performance is most likely to be its best.

Rituals make things happen that could otherwise not happen so easily or predictably. They involve manifesting power and therefore call for impeccable attention to their design and performance to ensure that the desired results are obtained and power is not abused.

In contrast to other cultures, modern Western society was largely devoid of rituals that move people into altered states of consciousness until the late 1960s, when people began experimenting with altered states of being to expand and explore human potential. Since then, people have flocked to various seminars and workshops, and many have discovered for the first time new states of transcendence, feeling, and being, with both positive and negative consequences. There is a serious need to develop critical thinking skills to evaluate these processes.[6] There are also three serious criticisms of some of the "new age" or human-potential movement "trainings" that need to be presented, because they have had a significant impact on society and the potential for forming a viable human community in harmony with itself and with nature.

While many promises may be made about relationships, communication, or even enlightenment, often very little of the information actually offers a planned, purposeful program to connect people with nature. Instead, participants are more often led through exercises that subtly and not so subtly seek to align people with the mental process of the leader, often using group hypnosis. When you bond with nature, you step into line with your ancestors and work toward individuation. When you bind with a leader on a transpersonal level, you run the risk of giving up personal identity and becoming part of a group mindfield that may not have your values. Graduates of such a process frequently come out feeling high and recruit others to join them, which is how the leaders of their programs make money. The graduates then become agents for the leaders and often develop a strong dependence on the group to maintain their identity.

My personal and professional experience has been that all too often trainings that make people dependent become a disruptive force in human community, rather than one that nourishes community synergy. Some of the leaders derive their identity from antagonizing the prevailing culture. Thus, graduates come out feeling superior and spend their time aggressively trying to get everyone else to be trained like them or disrupting existing systems just to vent pent-up feelings usually associated with powerlessness. In nearly every large event I've produced, people from some of these trainings have attempted to take over the event, as if on a holy war for their particular system. A good training, it seems to me, ought to make people more tolerant of others, compassionate, and able to work with anyone more easily, regardless of their background.

If I'm going to align myself with a teaching-healing force, I will put a lot more trust in caves, mountains, springs, owls, eagles, bears, buffalo, trees, and raccoons than human sharks. To prevent takeovers by power elites, I've borrowed an ancient technique from my shaman teachers. At the beginning of any event, I go out with key people in the project and conduct a ceremony at a special place, asking for guidance for the production of the event. Then, throughout the production process, we periodically renew this connection. People should use whatever they feel comfortable with to do this. Sincerity of intention, some type of sacrifice, and performing acts of service are the most important elements of right ritual and its application to generating community.

Some of these groups function as secret societies, kept that way through the use of special hypnotic inductions. Secret societies are an important part of human society, allowing for feelings of deep kinship. If you want to join a special group, why not consider some of the good ones that already exist, such as the Shriners or Masons, or even such groups as the Jaycees, Rotarians, Boy and Girl Scouts, and so on, all of which do notable community service work without muscling anyone into joining them and also have components that align people with nature.

Modern society tends to focus consciousness on a very small domain of the total realm of human potential. This makes us good at harmonizing with machines but stifles us emotionally and spiritually. Groups can make people go through states they didn't believe were possible. When this happens, because of our naïveté about altered states, people can come to believe that somehow the group is all-powerful. It isn't; it's only a tool. There are many ways to have transcendental experiences—isolation, fasting, near-death experiences, ordeals, dancing, making love, meditation, martial arts, praying, and so on. Groups are amplifiers and, for the most part, nonspecific amplifiers, which means that being in one, especially if you are sensitive, can resemble playing Russian roulette with your mind. As a therapist and teacher of therapists, I have seen and heard stories of hundreds of people who have suffered long-lasting, sometimes permanent, damage from being "trained." If you are one of these people who has been transported into realms you didn't expect or want to get into and are having difficulty, I encourage you to contact the Spiritual Emergence Network, an international referral system of therapists who are skilled in dealing with altered states. (See the Appendix for details.)

If you're going to journey into such a primeval territory as the wilderness of the mind, you ought to have a reliable guide, in this case a shaman. Shamans become guides because they have been through the states themselves, during a long, arduous apprenticeship program with seasoned teachers. It is their job to lead altered-state ceremonies. Also, shamans derive their power from intimate kinship bonding with nature. If you are well bonded with nature, wherever you go you will never be alone.

Shamans are not licensed or regulated; that would be impractical. But it might be appropriate for people who lead consciousness trainings to be required to put their credentials on permanent public record. For some kinds of events, licensed health professionals should be present.

A good training should make people more independent and self-reliant. Rather than leading people through exercises to generate emotional catharsis (which frequently serves the leader's ego more than the participants'), and then, while they are in an open, vulnerable state, asking them to sympathize with the leader's mind, the training ought to give people tools and techniques they can continue to use on their own. One of the greatest compliments I've ever received from someone who has used the methods I have presented here came from a man who confessed to me that he had seriously considered killing his spouse in the heat of passion. He knew no one to whom he could tell this, but he realized that nature is objective and created his own vision quest to determine if he should commit murder. Alone in the woods he sought to make contact with the animals, trees, rocks, and stars, which he had come to know were his allies and friends. As a result of renewing these connections, he had a powerful dream showing him his life's future and what he would miss out on in jail if he killed the person he hated. He emerged from the woods

with a smile on his face and a much deeper understanding of who
he was.

UNIFYING YOUR COMMUNITY BY
CREATING A SPIRIT OF PLACE

Novelist Tom Robbins recently remarked that "it's getting
harder to go anyplace in this world that has its own identity."
Part of the identity of any community is finding symbols that
bring it together and move it to environmental action. People
tend to think of Marin County as a place where everyone has a
hot tub, a BMW, and a handful of peacock feathers. Some of my
neighbors do, but not that many. Marin County is a lot like
many other parts of the country, including having a problem
with its solid-waste disposal. The citizens of Marin generate
garbage at the rate of 34 tons an hour, 822 tons a day, and 300,000
tons a year. If you took all of Marin's solid waste and dumped
it into Candlestick Park, where the 49ers play, at the end of the
year the whole park would be filled to within ten feet of the top.

Since 1985 half the landfills in the United States have been
closed, and the same is true for Marin's. Only one landfill—
quickly filling up San Francisco Bay—remains open to Marin's
garbage. Fortunately Marin is blessed with one of the nation's
best recycling programs, a weekly curbside pickup of paper,
glass, and cans by trucks with three separate compartments. As
of 1990, 25 percent of Marin's solid waste is being recycled, but
that's not enough. Since the technology is in place to recycle all
of Marin's recyclable materials, human cooperation is all that's
needed to stop filling up San Francisco Bay and to make trash
collection a very profitable business.

In the spring of 1990 my own organization, the Institute for
the Study of Natural Systems, working in cooperation with
Marin Solid Waste Management and Resource Recovery Association and a local community mental-health organization, the

Campaign for a Healthier Community for Children, sponsored a countywide art contest for children in grades K through 12 asking them to submit pictures of a recycling mascot for Marin County. A first prize of a weekend trip for four to Disneyland was donated by the local garbage-collection companies, and Marin World Africa-USA donated free passes to runners-up in the elementary, middle school, and high school divisions.

One thing Marin County has plenty of is creative people. Our judges were a head of a division of Lucasfilms' Oscar-winning Industrial Light and Magic (ILM), a nationally known sculptor-painter, and a representative of the solid-waste-collection agencies. We had 350 entries pour in. I was expecting the judges to choose one of the many sea gulls, raccoons, vultures, worms, pigs, goats, and crows that were submitted. To my amazement they unanimously agreed on a drawing by an eight-year-old boy of a man made entirely from trash.

Recycleman's head is a three-gallon garbage pail with a tin can on the top. His pendulous nose is a kitchen whisk, and his eyebrows are made from steel wool and copper scouring pads. His body is an old cardboard box that once held an electric guitar. The arms and legs are made from bits and pieces of junk, and the giant right hand has fingers made from toilet-paper inner tubes. He looks a little like the Tin Man from *The Wizard of Oz*, but his character is that of a rock-and-roll musician, crusading to promote recycling with humorous songs and rhymes. His special instrument is the "can do," which looks like a wizard's staff and contains an incredible collage of cans and a metal washboard on which Recycleman creates lively rhythms.

The original drawing of Recycleman was brought to life as a costume designed and built by Camilla Henneman and her associates in the Creature Department of Industrial Light and Magic. They have given us many modern mythic beings including Slimer, the Ewoks, and the other wondrous entities of the *Star Wars* trilogy. The many pieces of Recycleman's body came from the scrap pile at ILM, with glitter, glue, fabric, and so forth, and materials purchased with a grant from the Smith and Hawken company.

Emmy Award–winning songwriter Rita Abrams and I then penned Recycleman's first ballad, "The Recycling Blues," and he made his debut as an opening act for Jesse Colin Young at the 1990 Marin Earth Day celebration—with me inside, since another hat I wear is that of a musician and actor. To remind people that "the best things in life are biodegradable," Recycleman now appears with a band, Recycleman and the Collectors, who have opened for major rock bands and appeared on national television. In April 1991, Recycleman appeared on the floor of the California State Assembly to receive a special award for community service and leadership, following in the footsteps of the California Raisins and Walt Disney's characters.

Not every community would have chosen Recycleman as an environment mascot, but every community could use their own version of Recycleman to serve as an inspiration for new myths and symbols of ecological quality, and to help kids feel they have a role in creating an environmental ethic.

CREATING MODERN ECOLOGICAL FESTIVALS

Starting with rock concerts in the 1960s, making conferences, festivals, expositions, workshops, and concerts happen has been a major part of my life. Drawing on this experience, I've distilled what seem to be the basic elements of creating events that link people and nature together into an ecologically responsible community:

1. Each event has a "personality," which is the collective expression of the producers, the participants, and the place. The strength and clarity of this personality is usually a good indicator of the event's potential for success.
2. The success of the event (in terms of generating good, lasting

community spirit as well as money) is related to its ability to understand its people and its place. You will probably not draw many people to a winter fishing carnival in a community of vegetarians. The most successful events resonate with the needs and desires of the people one hopes to attract, not necessarily those values you personally hold dear. Many new ecology events are too righteous and fail to appeal to people who are not as deeply committed to eco-action ideals. Saul Alinsky, the master organizer of our times, always used to say that you've got to work with people where they're at, not where you're at or where you want them to be.

3. The most spiritually powerful events arise from the unique manifestations of nature in the lives of people who attend them. Agricultural festivals always tend to be popular when they can showcase the unique products and lifestyles of people who work directly with nature in creative ways. Natural landforms, unusual weather, or plant or animal life of a region will tend to draw people together much better than generic-theme events, unless you've got some big-name celebrities. The core sentiments for building an ecologically sustainable future will originate from tapping into the unique spirit of each place.

4. The most revitalizing events for a community allow for periods of license, when normal behavioral standards are set aside and people can safely enter into what in India is called the other mind, or, in Sanskrit, *anya-manas.* Common techniques include wearing costumes, holding parades, reversing community roles (having the mayor sweep the streets), holding street dances, and—in this age of ecology—closing down streets to cars. This allows people to vent pent-up feelings. The key to success is to know ahead of time what the unspoken feelings of the times are and to structure the freedom so that people learn to transmute negative energies into creative acts, not destructive or self-destructive ones. At the 1970 ENACT Teach-In we had a "car bash," in which participants paid to

take a swing with a sledgehammer at an old auto (thereby helping to fund the events). The feelings that were vented in the demise of that car could easily have leaked out into some people's attacking actual cars in protest at Detroit's sluggish response to environmentalists.

5. Festivals can influence social norms in two important ways: preserving and advancing certain cultural values, and offering opportunities for new ideas to surface and be evaluated. Because festivals are temporary environments that can be designed to display new ideas and behaviors, every modern festival should be a model of good ecological behavior through such things as recycling solid wastes, avoiding non-recyclable materials, and encouraging people to conserve resources with an ecologically sound set design. They should be places to set new standards and inspire creativity, glimpses of utopia.

6. The symbols, decoration, and pageantry used in creating the environment of the place can transform the setting for the performance into a mythic world of numinous symbols. At the 1989 Celebration for Mother Earth concert in Grace Cathedral in San Francisco, which I produced, while Bill Fields was narrating the Hopi creation myth of Spider Grandmother guiding the earth to life, we gently lowered an 8-foot-long purple spider made of balloons from the 200-foot-plus dome of the cathedral to the floor. When the spider disappeared behind the altar, a dancer dressed as Spider Grandmother emerged from the other side of the altar to depict her setting foot on earth. Then, going around the compass from each of the four directions came a procession of ten to twelve people moving to music pertaining to the direction. Each direction was also represented by colored banners, indigenous peoples of the world, and a costumed animal symbolic of that direction—a bear in the north, a whale in the west, a cougar in the south, and an eagle in the east.

7. The development of a festival entails a progression of many

ritual acts, each of which takes on more meaning by becoming part of a much greater whole. To heighten the experience and deepen its ecological teaching potential, you can do certain things during the process of preparation for the event that jar your perceptual process. One example is to hold "ecological fasts" for things we take for granted, such as electricity, water, gasoline, paper, watching television, and using wood products. Not using any one of these for a day will greatly change your appreciation of nature's presence and value in your life. Not speaking, reading, listening to the radio, or watching television for a day is a mind-expanding experience for many people, helping them shift into the ritual consciousness.

To begin planning an event, I always like to have people come together in a circle and go through a ritual process including saying why they are there. Then we light a white candle and make some kind of gesture of sacrifice—it could be sending clothing to needy Indian families or sprinkling some cornmeal at the foot of a tree—whatever seems appropriate. The white candle is based on my dream with the snow-geese people; we're requesting their presence and guidance in planning the event.

8. Call it good karma if you like, but I like to have every event I produce perform an act of service for some worthy cause. Over the years some of the events have given such services as picking up litter, planting trees, removing noxious plants from a national park, sending leftover food to the homeless, making donations to save the rain forests, gathering clothing to send to needy Indian tribes, and wheeling concrete and bricks for the construction of a Buddhist peace pagoda.

9. Any large event—festivals, conferences, expositions, and even rock concerts—can be a ritual filled with myths and symbols that encourage nature kinship—if the performers involved are willing to accept that they are ritualists and shamans. Mickey Hart, longtime drummer for the Grateful Dead rock band, has written a wonderful book, *Drumming at the Edge of*

Magic, which describes his own evolution toward understanding the spirit of the drum. His quest led him to many tribal shamans, as well as anthropologists and mythologists, bringing him to conclude that rock and roll can be an act of high shamanism. Mickey's ideas are shared by other members of the band, and Grateful Dead concerts are frequently filled with mythic symbols and ritual and spiritual elements in music and setting, sometimes including spiritual leaders in the programs, such as Tibetan monks and Indian medicine men. The feature film *The Doors,* about the life of the late rock star Jim Morrison, is a good case study of the making and breaking of an entertainer who was really a shaman but never fully surrendered to the responsibilities of having a spiritual calling. Effective rituals must be appropriate to the times, places, and people to whom they are offered.

These suggestions are offered as guidance on recovering the power of ritual to promote ecological values. Blend them with your creative ideas and the spirit of the place and develop an alchemy that makes the gods of nature come to life and reminds people what right livelihood is by means of wonder, awe, and joy.

TRANSLATING RITUALS INTO DESIGN STRUCTURES

The first environmentalists were the shamans, wizards, geomancers, dervishes, yogis, and witches, who went out into wild places to seek direct communion with the gods by striving to enter transpersonal states of consciousness. From these states they perceived sacred forms—some simple, such as the circle, triangle, and square, and others complicated, such as mandalas and mazes. These symbols and forms often become striking art of all forms, and they can also be used in architecture and design to ground the spiritual in the material, linking humans, nature, and spirit together in the sacred art and science of design.

Architecture and design today are all too often mechanical processes that are more based on ego, convenience, and economics
than on spirit and the land. The shapes that people enclose
themselves in influence their thinking and health. Just to illustrate the potentials that go unused for architecture to heal the
person-nature split, in American Samoa the mascot of Samoana
High School is the sea turtle, and its gymnasium is built in the
shape of a giant turtle, not the conventional box.

We are seeing more and more examples of planned neighbor-
hoods and communities with more green space. Some communities are hiring landscape architects such as Lawrence Halprin to
make parks that bring the feeling of wilderness into the city, the
way his Freeway Park in Seattle transports North Cascade
waterfalls to cover over an urban freeway or the way Levi-Strauss
Plaza in San Francisco offers a high-Sierras meadow to pass-
ersby. Adding more vegetation and waterfalls to cityscapes has
been shown to be valuable to community mental health as well
as to beautification. But what about the buildings! We desper-
ately need new kinds of structures to heal the perceptual split
between people and nature that is fostered by modern architecture.

Just a few miles outside of Kalamazoo, Michigan, is an example of an extraordinary building specially designed to link people
with the site on which it is built as well as with the universe—the
Fetzer Institute.

Born in 1901, John Earl Fetzer cultivated an early love of the
Marconi wireless (radio) and became a pioneer in broadcast
communications, inventing the directional antenna and becoming owner of many radio and television stations in the Midwest,
as well as eventually owning the Detroit Tigers baseball team.
Along the way Fetzer became fascinated by the concept of
subtle, invisible energies that influence health, partially because
of his work with energy fields. There had been occasions when
he healed himself of serious illnesses for which conventional
medicine had given him little time to live. In 1983 he sold his

franchise for the Detroit Tigers and set out on a bold new venture, to establish a research institute for the study of "energy medicine," which could bring together mind, body, spirit, and nature into a dynamic whole through applying state-of-the-art technologies to what he called the frontier science.

Fetzer believed that the building to house such a venture must be an expression of its philosophy. Investing an estimated fifteen million dollars, Fetzer used the best of ancient and modern knowledge about healthy buildings to create a "twenty-first-century center," which opened in 1987. The 57,000-square-foot administration building of the Fetzer Institute is set beside Dustin Lake in the gently rolling wooded countryside just west of Kalamazoo. The two-story building is in the shape of a triangle, the universal symbol of the mind. As you drive into the parking lot, cars circle a thirty-foot-tall stone-faced obelisk, which shields the building's cooling tower and reminds us of man's quest to contact God.

The design of the building is planned to make it "serve as a sanctuary of sanity." The color scheme of the granite building is inspired by the pyramids of Egypt, and as you enter, you walk under a giant Egyptian symbol of Thoth, the guide figure. The entrance walkway and floors are black, representing the physical plane. A dark-red granite arch (red symbolizing the mind) welcomes visitors into a two-story-high sunlit lobby containing a story-high, fifty-foot-long cascading waterfall surrounded by lush plant life and spectacular art objects. The roof and top of the atrium are white, symbolizing the spiritual realm.

The individual rooms are tastefully decorated with terrazzo floors, natural fibers and fabrics, polished brass fixtures that subtly suggest esoteric meanings, and woods from around the world. There is a special gymnasium and a cafeteria that serves tasty natural meals. To make the space extraordinarily healthy for people to work in and visit, sophisticated technologies have been used that include balanced, bipolar negative-air-ion generators in each room; incandescent- and fluorescent-shielded UV color-balanced lighting; reverse-osmosis-purified drinking water; fully shielded electrical wiring; and special sound insulation. The focal point of the institute is a meditation room with a seven-foot selenite crystal.

Aside from the inspiring feeling one gets walking through the building, I understand that the environmental-field controls are so good that it wasn't necessary to dust in the first two years that the building was open.

Some thirty people work at the Fetzer Institute, which is connected with a global network of scientists through a powerful computer system. Their mission is to facilitate science's moving into a new paradigm that will save the living earth and its human passengers. You may have designed the building differently if it were yours, but John Fetzer has made a statement that modern science and ancient wisdom can work together to solve mankind's problems. In addition to the work done at the Fetzer Institute, the building itself serves as an inspirational model, reminding us that we cannot afford not to think boldly if we want to create a sustainable society in the years to come. (Address of the Fetzer Institute appears in the Appendix.)

RETURNING TO GRACE

The ecological crisis we now face is a systemic problem, arising from the collective results of the many ways in which we have forgotten to know nature as an intimate friend. Like a marriage gone stale, when two people become too preoccupied with their own lives to stop and share with each other, things have gotten to the point where serious help is needed to restore the fondness that was once there. Modern science can agree with ancient wisdom that nature can and should be a teacher and healer in our lives. All signs point to acceptance of this attitude as essential to our survival. There is no amicable divorce possible between mankind and the earth in the forseeable future. Space travel to other planets is very far off.

The arguments and suggestions presented in this book lead one down a path. This path was once abandoned because it was feared that Satan or the devil lived at the end of it and that we would surely perish if we went that way. Now we know this is not true. Rather, the present path we are on—reducing the only acceptable model of reality to something provable by conventional mathematics and physics, separating the direct personal experience of spirit from the forms of religious practice, giving up using our senses as a basis for knowing the truth, and blindly following mechanical routines instead of engaging in life-affirming rituals charged with awe—leads to the land of the real demon who can kill us.

If we can return to the path of feeling we set aside when we went along with the assertion that nature kinship was useless superstition, we will find that the journey is worth the effort. Those who have made this journey understand. They know that following the path of wonder, humility, and awe—learning to listen with the third ear, the heart, to nature's guidance—will lead to the state of nature kinship that the Salish tribe calls *skalalitude.* In another tongue you might also call it love.

Restoring the magic of love for nature begins with each of us remembering what that love feels like. In addition to the things you may be doing now to help the ecology, consider making a special visit to a place in nature that seems to call you. It may be in a distant country or it may be a large tree right around the block. What's important is your motivation.

This place should have a special reverence for you. Approaching it should be like visiting a cathedral or a shrine. If it is a place with a long-standing use as a sacred place by an Indian tribe, stop along the way and buy something from a member of that group or send off a little money to an organization working to preserve the cultural heritage of traditional cultures.

As you arrive at the place, make a small offering of food, just a few grains of cornmeal. Drop them beside the path and explain to the place why you are there and what you hope to accomplish.

Quietly explore the area until you come to a place that seems to draw you to it. At that place, again make a little offering and then sit quietly. Watch, look, listen. Pray if you like, although stillness itself is a gesture of respect. Try to spend at least four to five hours at this place. During this time do not read, play music, or do anything else that will distract you from your attention to just being there. You can bring along a pad and some pencils to write or draw with. When you leave, pick up any litter you find. Leave the place cleaner than when you arrived.

Don't expect anything to happen, but be thankful if your pilgrimage is rewarded. When you achieve new levels of greater unity within yourself and harmony with nature, these connections will cause things to happen far beyond your own immediate personal experience—when you toss a pebble into the water, the waves may travel for a long time. Remember, too, the old saying that you don't always get what you want, but when you are connected with a higher purpose and seek the wise guidance of nature, you get what you need.

May the spirits of places you love always be with you, and you with them.

RESOURCES

NATURE GUIDES

Three of my favorite nature-guide writers are John Brainerd, Tom Brown, and Richard Nelson. Their books include:

Brainerd, John. *The Nature Observer's Handbook.* Chester, Conn.: Globe Pequot Press, 1986. A delightful guide to nature, written so that you can see the world through the eyes of a wise and witty naturalist. Read this book and new meanings will crop up all around you when you take a walk or go on a camping trip.

Brown, Tom. *The Tracker.* New York: Berkeley, 1978. Autobiographical; tells how to become a tracker as a life path; fascinating reading.

————. *Field Guide to Nature Observation and Tracking.* New York: Berkeley, 1983. Excellent guide by one of the best at outdoor lore today.

Nelson, Richard. *Make Prayers to the Raven: A Koyukon View of the Northern Forest.* Chicago: University of Chicago Press, 1983. A natural-history guide to Alaska as seen through the eyes of a Koyukon Indian wise person.

NATURAL HEALING

Two magazines that are very helpful resources for reading more about health and healing are *American Health* and *Prevention,* both of which are strong advocates of organic foods, proper diet, exercise, and nature appreciation.

Some books that are especially good include:

Bricklin, Mark. *The Practical Encyclopedia of Natural Healing.* Emmaus, Pa.: Rodale Press, Inc., 1976. A well-written, thorough encyclopedic treatment of natural-healing methods.

Brugh, Joy. *Joy's Way.* Los Angeles: J. P. Tarcher, Inc., 1979. Written by a physician, this is both autobiographical and extremely informative, showing how natural sensitivity can lead to health and healing.

Christopher, John. *The School of Natural Healing.* Provo, Utah: Biworld Publishing, 1976. An especially good book on herbalism and its use for all kinds of illness by the master of modern herbalism.

Eaton, S. B., M. Shostak, and M. Konner. *The Paleolithic Prescription.* New York: Harper & Row, Inc., 1989. The only diet book worth reading, this is based on an anthropological survey of human history, asking what has worked, not what a controlled study says.

Nixon, Frances. Frances Nixon has passed away, but her work continues to be carried on by more and more people. For details write to: Vivaxis Energies Research Society, 1525 West Seventh Avenue, Vancouver, B.C., Canada V6J 1S1.

Siegel, Bernie. *Love, Medicine and Miracles.* New York: Harper & Row, Inc., 1986. The modern classic story of healing, with special emphasis on attitude and self-healing.

Swan, James. *The Power of Place: Sacred Ground in Natural and Human Settings.* Wheaton, Ill.: Quest Books, 1991. An anthology based on the 1988 and 1989 "Spirit of Place" programs.

———. *Sacred Places: How the Living Earth Seeks Our Friendship.* Santa Fe, N.M.: Bear and Co., 1990. The value of sacred places in nature to modern and traditional cultures and the legal issues involved.

Taylor, Pat Ellis. *Border Healing Woman: The Story of Jewel Babb.* Austin, Tex.: University of Texas Press, 1982. A very well written story of a woman's discovery of her shamanic healing powers and the magic of Indian Hot Springs.

NATURE SOLO OPPORTUNITIES

An extended solo in nature is not for everyone, but if you feel you'd like to do this or participate in a more primal nature-bonding experience, the following people do good work and have a spiritual perspective:

Animas Valley Institute, 2655 W. Second Ave., Durango, Colo. 81301. Solos and small-group experiences in the beautiful Rocky Mountains of southwestern Colorado, led by seasoned psychologists and counselors with extensive wilderness experience.

Arctic Treks, Box 73452, Fairbanks, Alaska 99707. Carol Kasza and Jim Campbell are former Outward Bound instructors who lead ecologically conscious rafting and hiking trips into the Brooks Range and other Alaskan wilderness areas.

Brooke Medicine Eagle, Sky Lodge, P.O. Box 121, Ovando, Mont. 59854. Experiential programs along a Native American format led by Brooke, who has training in both ancient and modern healing methods.

Lewis Mehl, M.D., Resources for World Health, P.O. Box 42721, Tucson, Ariz. 85733 (602-647-3843). Lewis is a Cherokee physician who offers retreats combining modern psychology and traditional ceremonies.

Tom Pinkson, Ph.D., 240 Miller Avenue, Mill Valley, Calif. 94941. A clinical psychologist who leads wilderness solos in the Sierras.

Ojai Foundation, P.O. Box 5037, Ojai, Calif. 93023. A multifaceted educational center directed by anthropologist Joan Halifax.

Sacred Passage, Drawer CZ, Bisbee, Ariz. 85603. Wilderness solos in the Southwest guided by John Milton, who has an extensive background in natural resources and years of study of Buddhism.

For a more extended wilderness experience, the National Audubon Society Expedition Institute is a traveling, accredited school that offers a variety of programs for high school and college through master's-degree students. You travel the country in school buses, sleeping in sleeping bags and visiting Indians, Amish, back-to-the-earth people, and national parks for nine-month semesters, with a heavy emphasis on small-group process. Several solo experiences are offered during each semester. National Audubon Society Expedition Institute, P.O. Box 67, Mount Vernon, Me. 04352.

For information about wilderness trips led by the author, contact ISNS, P.O. Box 637, Mill Valley, Calif. 94942.

ENVIRONMENTAL MONITORING DEVICES

If you'd like to begin monitoring your own environment for noxious gases, electromagnetic-field pollution, radiation, and other subtle influences, a good source of inexpensive products and other energy-conserving devices is: Real Goods Trading Company, 966 Mazzoni Street, Ukiah, Calif. 95482 (800-762-7325).

ALTERNATIVES TO ANIMAL CRUELTY

A device that emits an ultrahigh-frequency sound from automobiles going over 35 mph that alerts animals to your approaching car is called the Animal Alert Safety Device. For information contact: Animal Alert, Inc., 2428 Southwest Ninth Street, Suite 4, Des Moines, Ia. 50315 (800-346-8316).

You can help stop unnecessary animal cruelty by buying health and cosmetic products that don't test their products on animals. A list of such companies can be obtained from In Defense of Animals, 21 Tamal Vista, Corte Madera, Calif. 94925.

FOR MORE INFORMATION...

Circle the Earth. Anna Halprin's productions are conducted by the Tamalpa Institute, P.O. Box 794, Kentfield, Calif. 94914. Information on Circle the Earth and other educational and training programs.

Feng Shui. Yun Lin Temple, 2959 Russell St., Berkeley, Calif. 94705. Quarterly newsletter is twenty dollars a year.

Fetzer Institute, 9292 West KL Avenue, Kalamazoo, Mich. 49009.

Ted Nugent's bowhunting magazine. *Ted Nugent's Bowhunter's World, Inc.,* P.O. Box 763, Grand Haven, Mich. 49417. Bimonthly, fifteen dollars a year. The most spirited outdoors magazine around!

Spiritual Emergence Network, 5905 Soquel Avenue, Suite 650, Soquel, Calif. 95073 (408-464-8261). International information and referral service for people going through spiritual crises.

AUDIOCASSETTES OF JOURNEYS DESCRIBED IN *NATURE AS TEACHER AND HEALER*

Audiocassettes of the guided-journey exercises described in this book can be purchased from the Institute for the Study of Natural Systems (ISNS), P.O. Box 637, Mill Valley, Calif. 94942. This is also the address for information about the "Spirit of Place" symposiums, Recycleman, and other projects by the author.

ASSISTANCE TO NATIVE AMERICANS

People ask for suggestions on how to help Native Americans. The Institute for the Study of Natural Systems works with two projects:

- Buffalo Restoration on Indian Lands. This project, directed by ISNS, seeks to restore buffalo herds on Indian reservations through musical concerts, gifts, grants, and sales of special products. Contributions and inquiries should be sent to ISNS at the address given above.
- Clothing Relief for the Lakota Reservations. The poorest county in the United States today is Shannon County, South Dakota, home of the proud Lakota Sioux tribe. Donations of warm clothing, over-the-counter medical supplies, and medical appliances should be sent directly to: Geraldine Janis, Community Health Representative Director, Oglala Sioux Tribe, P.O. Box A, Pine Ridge, S.D. 57770.

NOTES

INTRODUCTION: INSIDE-OUT ECOLOGY

1. Abraham H. Maslow, *The Farther Reaches of Human Nature* (New York: Viking Press, Compass Edition, 1971).

2. Thomas Tanner, "Significant Life Experiences: A New Research Area in Environmental Education," *Journal of Environmental Education,* Vol. XI, No. 4 (Summer 1980), pp. 20–24. And A. Sia, H. Hungerford, and A. Tomera, "Selected Predictors of Environmental Behavior," Department of Curriculum, Instruction, and Media, Southern Illinois University, Carbondale, Ill., 1984.

3. Gifford Pinchot, *Breaking New Ground* (New York: Harcourt, Brace and World, 1947), p. 40.

4. This research is described in *This World,* May 15, 1983, in the story "The We-Never-Rest Society" by Kent A. MacDougall.

5. Maslow, *The Farther Reaches,* p. 332.

CHAPTER ONE: RETURNING TO THE ROOTS

1. This theory is advanced by Frances Nixon in a number of her books, including *Mysteries of Mind Unfold* (Chemainus, British Columbia: Magnetic Publishers, 1979), and is confirmed by the personal experiences of thousands of people including myself and my family.

2. R. D. Vaughn and G. L. Harlow, "Findings—Report on the Pollution of the Detroit River, Michigan Waters of Lake Erie, and Their Tributaries" (Washington, D.C.: U.S. Department of Health, Education and Welfare, Public Health Service, 1965).

3. Carl Gustav Jung, *Civilization in Transition,* Vol. 10, *Collected Works of Carl Jung* (New York: Pantheon, 1964), p. 49.

4. Herbert Kelman, "Processes of Opinion Change," *Public Opinion Quarterly,* Vol. XXV (Spring 1961), pp. 55–78.

5. Aniela Jaffé, "Symbolism in the Visual Arts", Part IV in *Man and His Symbols,* ed. C. G. Jung (New York: Dell Publishing Co., 1968), p. 266.

CHAPTER TWO: LEARNING TO SURRENDER

1. Quoted in T. C. McLuhan, ed., *Touch the Earth* (New York: Promontory Press, 1973), p. 23.

CHAPTER THREE: DISSOLVING THE
FEAR OF NATURE

1. Carroll Izard, *Human Emotions* (New York: Plenum Press, 1977), p. 35.

2. I. M. Lewis, *Ecstatic Religion: An Anthropological Study of Spirit Possession and Shamanism* (New York: Penguin Books, 1971).

3. "Science Academy Says Chemicals Do Not Necessarily Increase Crops," *The New York Times,* September 8, 1989.

4. Marie-Louise von Franz, *Shadow and Evil in Fairy Tales* (Zurich: Spring Publications, 1974), p. 154.

5. Boyce Rensberger, *The Cult of the Wild* (Garden City, N.Y.: Anchor Press, Doubleday, 1977).

6. Franz Boas, *The Social Organization and Secret Societies of the Kwakiutl Indians,* Report of the U.S. National Museum, Washington, D.C., 1895; and Peter Macnair, "Kwakiutl Winter Dances: A Reenactment," in *Stones, Bones and Skin: Ritual and Shamanic Art,* eds. Anne Trueblood Brodsky, Rose Danesewich, and Nick Johnson (Toronto: Arts Canada, 1977), pp. 62–82.

CHAPTER FOUR: ECOLOGICAL GUILT

1. Friends of Animals, *Hunting—An Act Against Nature* (New York: Friends of Animals, n.d.), p. 1.

2. Steven Kellert's research is described in detail in John Mitchell's excellent book *The Hunt* (New York: Knopf, 1976), p. 20.

3. José Ortega y Gasset, *Meditations on Hunting* (New York: Scribner's, 1972).

4. *Ibid.*

5. Richard K. Nelson, "The Gifts," in *On Nature: Nature, Landscape and Natural History*, ed. Daniel Halpern (San Francisco: North Point Press, 1987), p. 117.

6. Danny Slomoff, "Ecstatic Spirits: A West African Healer at Work," *Shaman's Drum*, No. 5 (Summer 1985), pp. 27–31.

7. Franz Boas, *The Religion of the Kwakiutl Indians*, vol. Z: Translations (New York: Columbia University Press, 1930), p. 619.

8. Ted Nugent, "Ted Nugent's World Bowhunters By-Laws," *Ted Nugent's World Bowhunters Magazine*, Vol. 2, No. 1, (Dec. 1990/Jan. 91), p. 9.

9. *Ibid.*, p. 31.

10. Jimmy Carter, *An Outdoor Journal: Adventures and Reflections* (New York: Bantam, 1988), p. 5.

CHAPTER FIVE: NATIVE AS TEACHER

1. Aldo Leopold, *A Sand Country Almanac* (New York: Oxford University Press, 1966), p. 239.

2. *Ibid.*, p. 240.

3. *Ibid.*, p. 130.

4. *Ibid.*, p. 239.

5. Richard Nelson, *Make Prayers to the Raven: A Koyukon View of the Northern Forest* (Chicago: University of Chicago Press, 1983), p. 14.

6. Thomas Armstrong, *In Their Own Way* (Los Angeles: J. P. Tarcher, 1987).

7. Robert Graves, *The White Goddess* (New York: Farrar, Straus and Cudahy, 1948), pp. 16–21.

8. Lesley Gordon, *Green Magic: Flowers, Plants and Herbs in Lore and Legend* (New York: Viking Press, 1977).

9. Christopher Finch, *The Art of Walt Disney* (New York: Portland House, 1988 edition), p. 160.

10. Charles L. Woodward, *Ancestral Voice: Conversations with N. Scott Momaday* (Lincoln, Neb.: University of Nebraska Press, 1989).

11. Vine Deloria, Jr., "Land and Revelation," Keynote speech at the "Spirit of Place" Symposium, "Sacred Spaces and Places," Grace Cathedral, San Francisco, August 18, 1989.

CHAPTER SIX: NATURE AS HEALER

1. Theodore Roosevelt, *Theodore Roosevelt: An Autobiography* (New York: Macmillan, 1914), p. 14.

2. Lawrence LeShan, *The Mechanic and the Gardener* (New York: Holt, Rinehart & Winston, 1982), p. 16.

3. Quoted in Charles A. Ziegler, *Environmental Policy in the USSR* (Amherst, Mass.: University of Massachusetts Press, 1987), p. 10.

4. Robert O. Becker and Gary Selden, *The Body Electric* (New York: Quill, Morrow, 1985), p. 26.

5. "Soviet Science: A Wonder Water from Kazakhstan," *Science,* Vol. CCII (October 27, 1978), p. 414.

6. Robert Miller, "Paraelectricity: A Primary Energy," *Human Dimensions,* Vol. V, No. 1–2, Buffalo, N.Y. (n.d.), pp. 24–26.

7. Pat Ellis Taylor, *Border Healing Woman* (Austin, Tex.: University of Texas Press, 1981), p. 62.

8. Pat Ellis Taylor, *The God Chaser* (Austin, Tex.: Slough Press, 1986), pp. 180–182.

9. Norman Cousins, *Anatomy of an Illness as Perceived by the Patient* (New York: W. W. Norton, 1979), p. 48.

10. *World Research News,* 3rd and 4th quarters, 1989, p. 7.

11. Yukio Ishihara, "Today's Mental Health Care–Day Care of Mental Patients," *Byoin* (Tokyo), Vol. XXXII, No. 12 (1973), pp. 54–58.

12. Jean Achterberg, *Imagery and Healing: Shamanism and Modern Medicine* (Boston: Shambala Press, 1985).

13. *The Oakland Tribune,* February 5, 1986.

14. Kund Rasmussen, *Across Arctic America* (New York: G. P. Putnam and Sons, Inc., 1927), pp. 82–84.

15. This material is presented in Cousins, *Anatomy of an Illness.*

16. Richard Nelson, *Make Prayers to the Raven* (Chicago: University of Chicago Press, 1983), p. 45.

17. Bernie Siegel, *Love, Medicine and Miracles* (New York: Harper & Row, 1986), p. 49.

18. Kenneth Pelletier, *Mind as Healer, Mind as Slayer* (New York: Delta, 1978).

CHAPTER SEVEN: THE SPIRIT OF PLACE

1. Francis J. Newcomb and Gladys Reichard, *Sandpaintings of the Navajo Shooting Chant* (New York: Dover Publications, 1975), p. 69.

2. D. H. Lawrence, *Studies in Classical American Literature* (New York: Thomas Seltzer and Sons, 1923), pp. 8–9.

3. Christopher Alexander, *A Pattern Language* (New York: Oxford University Press, 1977), p. xvi.

4. The Geo Group can be contacted at P.O. Box 298, Mercer Island, Washington 98040.

CHAPTER EIGHT: PERSONAL POWER
AND NATURE

1. Rudolf Steiner, *An Outline of Occult Science* (Spring Valley, N.Y.: Anthroposophic Press, 1972), p. 28.

2. Rudolf Steiner, Lecture of September 28, 1921, *In Partnership with Nature* (Wyoming, R.I.: Bio-Dynamic Literature, 1981), p. 40.

3. Michael Murphy, "Afterword: Sport as Yoga," in *Beyond Jogging: The Innerspaces of Running* (Berkeley, Calif.: Celestial Arts, 1976), pp. 99–110.

4. Charles Tart, *States of Consciousness* (New York: E. P. Dutton, 1975).

5. David Wharton, "I Will Fear No Burning Coals on My Toes," *Los Angeles Herald Examiner,* May 7, 1983.

6. Natalie Curtis, *The Indians' Book: An Offering by the American Indians of Indian Lore, Musical and Narrative, from a Record of the Songs and Legends of Their Race* (New York: Harper & Row, 1907), p. 96.

7. Lama Anagarika Govinda, "Sacred Mountains," in W. Y. Evans-Wentz, *Cuchama and Sacred Mountains,* ed. Frank Waters (Chicago: Swallow Press, 1981), p. xxix.

8. Carlos Castaneda, *Journey to Ixtlan* (New York: Simon and Schuster, 1972).

9. W. C. Beane and W. G. Doty, *Myths, Rites and Symbols—A Mircea Eliade Reader* (New York: Harper Colophon, 1975), Vol. 1, p. 154.

10. Marghanita Laski, *Ecstasy: A Study of Some Secular and Religious Experiences* (Bloomington, Ind.: University of Indiana Press, 1961), p. 266.

11. David Foster, "Redford Using Star Status in Down-to-Earth Activism," New Orleans *Times-Picayune,* November 12, 1989, pp. A–9.

12. Gary Snyder, *The Old Ways* (San Francisco: City Lights, 1977), p. 56.

13. Marie-Louise von Franz, *Number and Time* (Evanston, Ill.: Evanston Press, 1974).

14. Elmer Green and Alyce Green, "Epilogue," in Doug Boyd, *Rolling Thunder* (New York: Delta, 1974), p. 272.

15. H. Ostermann, "The Alaskan Eskimos as Described in the Posthumous Notes of Dr. Knud Rasmussen." *Report of the Fifth Thule Expedition 1921–24,* Vol. X, No. 3 (Copenhagen, Denmark: Nordisk Forlag, 1952), p. 99.

16. Press release from Vail Associates, Inc., January 6, 1977.

17. *Rocky Mountain News,* November 4, 1989. Reported in *Shaman's Drum,* Midwinter 1990, p. 11.

18. Frank Waters, *The Man Who Killed the Deer* (Chicago: Swallow Press, 1942), p. 27.

CHAPTER NINE: KEEPING NATURE'S MAGIC IN YOUR LIFE

1. René Dubos, *The Wooing of the Earth* (New York: Scribner's Sons, 1980), p. 7.

2. Bill Moyers, *The Movement Action Plan* (San Francisco: The Movement for a New Society, 721 Shrader St., San Francisco, Calif. 94117), Spring 1987.

3. Joseph Campbell, *The Hero with a Thousand Faces* (Princeton, N.J.: Princeton/Bollingen Paperback edition, 1972), p. 236.

4. Chung-Liang Al Huang, *Quantum Soup* (New York: E. P. Dutton, 1983).

5. Rina Swentzell and Tito Naranjo, "Nurturing: The Gia at Santa Clara Pueblo," *El Palacio,* Vol. XCII, No. 1 (Summer–Fall 1986).

6. For further readings on possible dangers of human potential seminars and trainings see: Elmer Green and Alyce Green, *Beyond Biofeedback* (New York: Delacorte, 1977); Janice Haaken and Richard Adams, "Pathology as Personal Growth: A Participant-Observation Study of Lifespring Training," *Psychiatry,* Vol. XLVI (August 1983); Janice Haaken and Richard Adams, "Anticultural Culture: Lifespring's Ideology and Its Roots in Humanistic Psychology," *Journal of Humanistic Psychology,* Vol. XXVII, No. 4 (Fall 1987, pp. 501–517). Also see "Where Is Werner Erhard?" *San Francisco Examiner,* April 21, 1991, p. 1; "Werner Dearest," *Marin Independent Journal,* Lifestyles section, June 17 and 18, 1990, p. 1; and David Gelman, "The Sorrows of Werner: For the Founder of est, a Fresh Round of Charges," *Newsweek,* Feb. 18, 1991, p. 72.

INDEX

ABOUT THE AUTHOR

JAMES A. SWAN, Ph.D., is one of the founders of the modern field of environmental psychology. He is professor of anthropology at the California Institute of Integral Studies and co-director of The Institute for the Study of Natural Systems. He has previously taught at the University of Michigan, Western Washington State University, University of Oregon, and University of Washington in both environmental studies and psychology, and consulted on environmental education with many state and federal agencies and national organizations. Searching for answers to how traditional peoples live in harmony with nature has taken him from above the Arctic Circle to the South Pacific and all across the United States and Canada, working with Native Americans. His writing has appeared in many popular magazines and two recent books, *Sacred Places* and *The Power of Place.* His work has received recognition from the American Public Health Association, Psi Chi Psychology Honorary, The American Nature Study Society, and the California State Assembly. Dr. Swan is also an accomplished musician and actor, as well as a producer of concerts, expositions, and symposiums. The January 1, 1990, issue of the *San Francisco Examiner* called him "One of the 90 people to watch in the nineties."